# SPECIAL OPERATIONS FITNESS PREPARATION PROGRAM

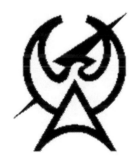

**....A-TAC THE WORLD....**

# Legal Notice

Copyright ® 2019 by A-TAC Fitness

All rights reserved. No part of this publication may be reproduced, distributed, or transmitted in any form or by any means, including photocopying, recording, or other electronic or mechanical methods, without the prior written permission of the publisher, except in the case of brief questions embodied in critical reviews and certain other noncommercial uses permitted by the copyright law. For permission requests, write to admin@atacfitness.com

www.atacfitness.com
ISBN: 978-1-7342855-0-5

## Disclaimer

The content provided in this book is designed to provide helpful information on the subjects discussed; it is not meant to be used or should it be used to diagnose or treat any medical condition. For diagnosis and treatment of any medical problem consult with your doctor, physician, or other qualified medical professional.

All material and any content contained on or in this book is for informational purposes only and is not intended to substitute the advice, diagnosis, or treatment from a qualified or licensed medical professional. Always consult with your doctor, physician, or other qualified medical professional with any medical questions you may have.

The publisher, the book or the writer does not make any representations, recommend or endorse any specific tests, products, procedures, opinions, or other information that is mentioned in or on this book. Additionally, we are not responsible for any specific health or allergy needs that may require medical supervision and are not liable for any damages or negative consequences for any treatment, action, application or preparation to any person reading or following the information in this book. Reliance on any information provided by A-TAC Fitness and its writer, Jonathon Castillo, is solely at your own risk.

We are not endorsed or associated with the United States Air Force, nor do we represent the opinions, views or any characterization that can be defined, of the United States Air Force. Any and all information contributed in this book is based solely on personal experience. Results are not typical and may vary per individual.

# Table Of Contents

**Mindset Conditioning** — 1
    Stop Giving Excuses — 2
    The Power Of Mindset — 4

**Recovery Diet** — 10
    What Is Protein? — 11
    What About Protein Powders? — 13
    Ways To Add More Protein In Everyday Diet — 14
    Planning Your Recovery Phase — 16

**Recovery & Performance Enhancing Supplements** — 18
    Significance of Muscle Gaining Supplements — 18
    Top 3 Muscle Gaining Supplements — 19
    Rule of Thumb for a Good Diet — 22
    Supplements To Avoid — 24
    Testosterone Booster — 24
    Protein Supplement Scams — 27

**A-TAC 8 Week Beginner Fitness Program** — 29

**Special Operations Fitness Preparation Program** — 39
    Phase 1 — 41
    Personal Assessment — 52
    Phase 2 — 54

**THAT OTHERS MAY LIVE – FIRST THERE**

# MINDSET
## CONDITIONING

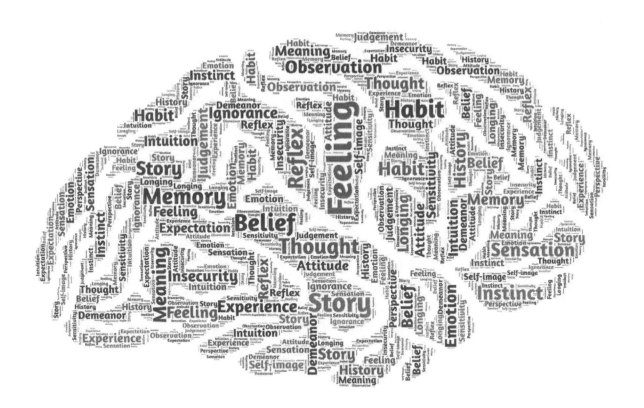

# Mind-set Conditioning

## Stop Giving Excuses

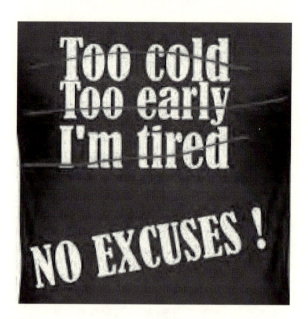

"You can have results or excuses. Not both."

Roadblocks, brick walls, obstacles, bumps in the road, reasons or whatever you call them - they exist and they get in our way daily, on our quest to become on the few spoken, the legends that everyone pretends they were, but never achieved.

Stop giving excuses. When you are out in the field you think an excuse is going to bring you home? You think that because you're not in a pool it's different? No…You will BREAK and HAVE a FULL-BLOWN MENTAL BREAKDOWN as the water touches you. Do you think I'm making this up? I saw it myself... On the bus ride there it started, he poisoned his mind... we geared up, his toe touched the water...and he broke... I quit!!! He stood up, right away, shaking. The funny thing was that it was a recovery day. The best way to get back on board is to stop making excuses.

Below I've provided the 5 most common excuses people have used to quit:

- I can't do it, this is too hard (cliché I know, but you would be surprised when hypoxia kicks in and you just want a little oxygen how often this is thought.)

- I have no motivation to wake-up (Motivation is trash, your drive is what matters, 3 AM you have to be downstairs ready to go, after your body is trashed.)

- I feel intimidated by the cadre there (Guess what? They all started just like you, they weren't a badass, they were trained to be one, exactly like you are right now.)

- I don't have anyone that relates (Clear out the water out of your mask, do you not see everyone struggling around you? Those are your brothers! No matter if you mess up, they will have your back, trust me I know.)

- I'm on a whole-body medical waiver (No, that's not a joke. Someone literally went on a whole-body waiver so they could say they didn't "Quit". If this isn't for you have the decency to say so, at least you will get the respect of your peers.)

These are some of the standard excuses for not making it that can be heard around recruiters and other places in the military. Those that have been there and done it will tell you none matter, it all came down to how badly you wanted it. Is it hard? Beyond a doubt. BUT… You CAN MAKE IT! Even Navy SEALS need to call 911 right? Do you think an average Joe will be cut out to aid the elite like a SEAL? So don't expect to get through it with an average mind.

To achieve this, you have to stop making excuses. Not just that, your mindset plays a significant role as well. A positive mindset is the most powerful tool for reaching and destroying obstacles. The way you perceive your journey will either make or break you.

# The Power Of The Mindset

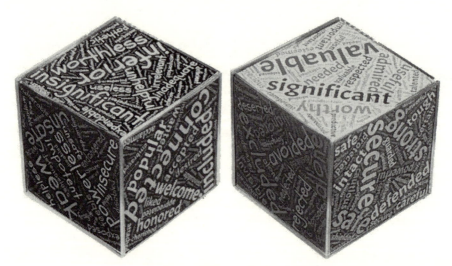

Becoming Phenomenal begins with the mind, not the body. Never underestimate the power of your mind. The mind has always been at the core of greatness. Clear all negative thinking and replace them with positive ones to empower you. You cannot just go ask an average person how to become great. If you ask an average person how do you become phenomenal, they are going to give you advice on how to be a great average person. This includes your mom, dad, friends etc. Understand that your thoughts are what hold you back from what you truly want to achieve. You have to see it before you even have it, it has to be real to you even if it's not real to those around you.

The essentiality of having a strong mind is often overshadowed by being strong physically. If you have the right mindset, you will have the mental power to stay focused and push yourself, even when things get tough. Not having the right mindset will result in you ending up sabotaging your dream.

So how do you 'Fix' your mindset? Here are 5 Simple Techniques to help you achieve your dream body with the right mindset:

## 1. Set Goals That Are Both Specific & Achievable (by achievable I don't mean average)

You CAN make it if you have a crystal-clear outcome. So, remember to always begin with the end in mind.

Ask yourself questions like: What would it feel like to wear my beret? How strong or fast do I need to become? Can I stay calm while everything is going wrong? Can I focus when someone's life hangs in the balance? Is my goal only attainable in three months or more? What is it going to take to achieve this job? The 2 Rules is to be both Specific & Achievable - do not just estimate or simply see-how-it-goes. Train exactly how the regimen is listed. Do the exact amount listed in the program later on. We took the guess work out for you, just grind like no other. We got the specific down for you, it's up to YOU to ACHIEVE it!

Without setting specific and achievable goals, you are more likely to stumble and fail. Make your goals specific, write them down! Then put your list of goals onto your mirror, your fridge, your work table, or even your phone screen - just anything that's clearly visible to you every day. This will keep you reminded of your most important goals every day whether you feel like it or not. In the long-term, this will condition your mind in an empowering way! Mindset conditioning has immense- power in fueling your determination and commitment.

## 2. Cultivate Patience

You need time to achieve your desired goals and this requires patience. Be patient for results because learning new techniques does not happen overnight. Take a step back and evaluate what you have achieved so far. Cultivate patience and learn to celebrate little victories along the way in your goal-setting process. This will encourage and motivate you to keep you going.

Everybody is wired differently. So many people expect results in a minimal timeframe and then give up hope when what they are training for is nowhere to be seen. Nothing comes easily. Trust me on this one, it took me months to teach myself to swim, it was like learning to walk, just so I could pass the PAST.

Embarrassing myself in front of some fairly attractive girls, they were there teaching babies how to swim. The sad part is, I think the babies would have fared better than I at the time.

Just focus on the fundamentals and the rest will come. Eat smart, work hard, and most importantly have the patience for results. Remember that Rome wasn't built in a Day, and same with you. If you're working with the right Program like this one, eventually the results will prove to you all its worth.

## 3. Hard Work Is Your Only "Shortcut"

There really isn't any shortcut to being a PJ or a USAF Special Operator. The only "SHORTCUT" is seeking the right guidance, from tried and true information. The only way to expedite the process is to gather all the information into one place and use it. Luckily, we have done that for you, this is the "Shortcut" so all you have to focus on training and stop wasting your time looking for answers on the internet. If you do, you'll notice it is always a gradual process, you will start PAST test requirements, PJ workout guides eventually falling down the rabbit hole questioning why you started. How do I know this? Do you know how often it has been asked and searched, "What happens if I wash-out?". If this is a concern, then apparently you skipped over the mindset portion of this program. Those words should not even cross your mind. So this program has brought all the information you need into one place, keeping you from wasting time with meaningless research.

There is no substitute for hard work in fitness. The only thing you need to get started is the right knowledge, diet plan, and workout regime. From there, all you need is relentless hard work, patience, and determination to stay on track.

## 4. Everyone Is Different. Don't Compare

Do not compare yourself to others. Everyone is different – your body as well, what you are and what you do are different from other people.

I am a calisthenics freak, I also had more strength to my body than most people thought, I however, was not a strong swimmer or runner. Now I am not a slow runner or swimmer by any means, nor I am the fastest. I consider myself a good average swimmer and runner. People would smoke me in the run and swim, I was right in the middle and towards the end in the swim. However that did not deter me. If anything, I knew my weak spots and sprinted the last lap and throw up outside of the pool just to make the time.

This comparison is unnecessary, it brings disappointment and zero help towards your goal. Focus on your own strengths and weaknesses. Aim for incremental progress until you can finally keep up with others. Now this is not an excuse for you to half-ass something. Remember I mentioned that I would throw up outside of the pool once I was done? Well because I pushed myself to keep up with the rest, looking at it as a challenge, not as a boohoo pity party reason as to why I was not going to make it and they were. That's pathetic and you know it.

## 5. Be Completely Committed

This lifestyle is all about Discipline. The ability to consistently take action regardless of how you feel at any moment.

Commit yourself 100% for however many days it takes to get in and stay in. 2 weeks or 4 months. You shouldn't be deterred from the goal, if you are then you were never in it for real then.

This mindset helps you to be realistic. You won't be bogged down if you don't meet a run or swim time, you'll be focusing on the process and duration. Because you understand and are aware that you are a warrior, the elite, the grind is what you look forward to, the hunt… it takes time and effort. When you are mentally prepared to commit you will persevere through the process.

Here are some strategies to keep you on track when the journey gets too bumpy:

Journaling - It helps you to track your own progress

Progress videos – This tremendous for watching your swim technique, after all swimming is all technique.

Training Buddy - Mental and physical support play a big role in helping you make it through the pipeline. _This, however can be a double edge sword. IF your buddy were to quit. THIS could mess with your head and your confidence._

**THAT OTHERS MAY LIVE – FIRST THERE**

# RECOVERY DIET

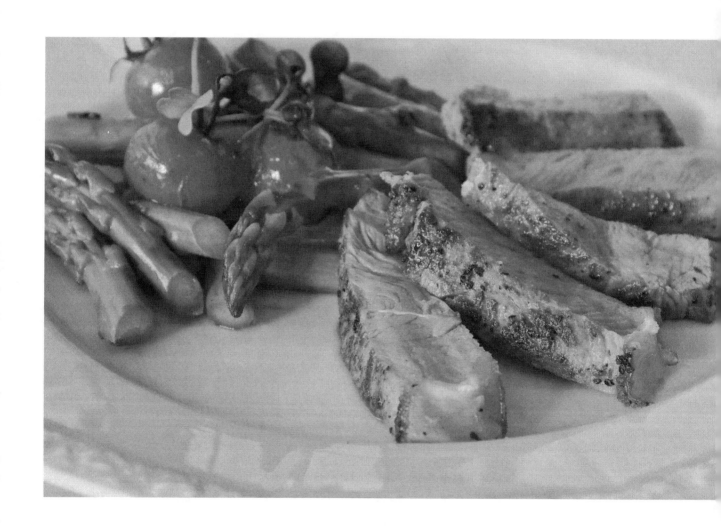

# Recovery Diet

There are many gurus that swear by high-protein diets such as Zone, Atkins and Sugar Busters to get in shape, they are far from what you're trying to reach. Following any of these diets while training at elite levels has one alarming flaw; unbalanced meals, this will deprive your body of other essential nutrients needed to recover. However, that doesn't have to be the case.

High protein diets are generally suitable for individuals looking to burn fat and lose weight with a caloric deficit. If you are training to be an elite athlete there you need to consume a mixture of proteins, carbohydrates and fats. Carbohydrates supply you with energy to blast those weights in the gym and also fill in the caloric surplus you need to actually maintain weight and build muscles (trust me this is a must, I have never met anyone that has gained weight through selection, selection is designed to break your body down.) Furthermore, studies show that diet rich in carbs, protein and fats can help maintain energy levels while building muscle, especially in tactical athletes.

## What Is Protein?

Protein is one of the 3 main macronutrients along with carbohydrates and fat. Protein is the most important source for muscle gaining as it acts as building blocks for muscle fibers. Simply said, without protein, your muscles won't be able to grow. The best sources of protein are lean meat, eggs, cottage cheese, beans, quinoa and many others. We called these foods 'Protein-rich

Powerfoods' as they are packed with a higher percentage of protein compared to other nutrients.

To have a better understanding of what protein really is, it is a large molecule composed of smaller units known as the amino acids. Today, we can identify 20 types of amino acids. Different types of proteins are actually derived from different combinations of amino acids. This essential macronutrient can be found in any part of the human body. Your organs, hair, skin, nails, eyes, nose, lips are all made up of protein.

Ultimately, there will be no muscle gain without protein.

## What Foods Contain High Amounts Of Protein?

Working out involves breaking down muscle fibers in order to grow bigger and stronger, protein is NEEDED to repair and grow these muscle fibers. Also, it's good to note that protein is the final source of energy after both carbohydrates and fats are depleted, this is the reason you want to upkeep your carbs and fats. Preventing a decline in performance.

Protein is available from both animal and plant sources. The typical U.S. diet is a mixture of protein sources. A variety of choices will provide an adequate diet. The following are some examples of protein content in some typical foods.

- 3oz. of chicken contains 20g of protein
- 3 oz. of ground beef contains 21g of protein

- 2 oz. of pork chop contains 15g of protein
- ¾ cup of beans contains 11g of protein
- 2 tablespoons of peanut butter contain 8g of protein
- ½ cup of soybeans contains 10g of protein

## What About Protein Powders?

Speak to any fitness enthusiasts in the gym, you'll find that most of them consume protein powders and it is their holy grail of supplements.

So, what exactly are they?

It's actually a popular protein source to help people improve athletic performance and build muscle mass. This is a go-to solution for those who are looking for a quick and convenient source to fill in their daily protein intake requirements and aid in recovery. Generally, one scoop of protein powder contains about 25g of protein, and 2 scoops can easily make up with one chicken breast. Plus, it's easier to chuck down a bottle of protein shake than digesting one whole chicken breast.

That said, protein powder is an excellent way to supplement your daily protein needs, especially if you're looking to train like a madman and still recover. Here are the types of proteins you can find in the market today:

1) **Whey Protein Concentrate** – The most common and affordable form of

whey protein. Most of them contain lactose. So for those who are lactose-intolerant, stay away from this.

2) **Whey Protein Isolate** – A more concentrated form of whey protein with little to no fat or lactose. This is the number one choice for those with lactose-intolerant and also the purest form of whey protein you can find today. Whey Protein Isolate usually contains zero carbohydrates and zero fats.

3) **Hemp Protein** – A plant-based protein. Perfect for vegans with additional anti-inflammation benefits from included Omega-3 fatty acids with extra fiber for weight loss and gut health.

4) **Pea Protein Powder** – Another plant-based protein. Vegans' favorite. Nothing necessarily special with this one, usually you can find this one on sale, but it's not as easily absorbed into the body like whey.

5) **Soy Protein Powder** – Just like whey protein, you can find them in concentrate and isolate form. This type of protein comes with a different taste and texture for consumers.

## Ways To Add More Protein In Everyday Diet

Besides protein powder, you should also learn how to get your protein intake from other sources, including whole food. Here's a list of food that you can consider adding into your everyday diet to hit your daily protein target:

**Cheese.** Preferably cheese with low fat and high protein such as string cheese. You can have them as snacks on the go or add them to your meals. Some even prefer to melt them on slices of bread and noodles or even grate and add them to mashed potatoes and their favorite meat for variety.

**Cottage cheese or ricotta cheese.** Another excellent source of casein protein, a slow-digesting protein that drip-feed your muscles for the entire day. You can consume them as is or even add them to your favorite fruits or vegetables for extra sweetness.

**Milk or soy milk.** Milk is considered to be an easy source of protein. Most milks contain high carbohydrates and fats.

**Yogurt.** This is a good choice for dessert. You can add yogurt to your favorite fruits, cereals, and high-protein snacks to create a wholesome, guilt-free snack.

**Eggs.** You can find some of the purest forms of protein from eggs. Top Bodybuilders over the decades swear by the benefits of consuming eggs daily. Also, eggs are the cheapest source of protein you can get out there and can be cooked in numerous ways. They can be hard-boiled, soft-boiled, scrambled, poached, pan-fried, baked, basted and sunny-side up. Really now, you can never go wrong with eggs. Careful though as your cholesterol CAN go up if you eat them whole. How do I know? Because even though some science says they can't, I ate 6 raw eggs every day for a year straight, non-stop. Got blood work done and my cholesterol was borderline a problem, however my performance did improve.

**Nuts, seeds, wheat germ, and oats.** These are the secret snacks you can consume for satiety and excellent protein and fat source. These power-foods contain so many benefits on top of being an excellent protein source.

**Meat and fish.** These are the biggest protein sources you can find to pack on some lean, mean muscle mass. However, if you're a vegan, consider other protein sources above such as nuts, quinoa, cheese and many others.

## Planning Your Recovery Phase

Tactical athletes who are attempting to add muscle and strength over time don't have the same macronutrient needs as bodybuilders and average gym-goers. They will be in a caloric surplus and most likely have a higher body fat percentage compared to bodybuilders. Why? Because you're after performance not looks, although you will develop quite a bit of muscle, there's no need to see every little striation on your back or quads.

As mentioned before, research shows that high protein intake doesn't necessarily guarantee straight performance. In fact, it is shown that you can have an anabolic effect of high protein diets doesn't extend past around 0.8-1.1 g/lb. Thus, it is recommended to consume 0.8-1.1 g/lb of protein on a daily basis to reap all the benefits of protein in your diet.

The rest of your diet should be filled with carbohydrates and fats to fill in the caloric gaps. Now this is a tricky one, because largely it depends on an individual's metabolism. While there is a general margin of 3-12 grams of carbs per kg of bodyweight. Where you fall in that you will need to assess on your own. However, if you are truly giving this program your all it wouldn't surprise me if you are closer to the end of this scale. But like mentioned before, this can vary per individual.

When planning your recovery diet plan, first decide how many calories you are burning, this is generally easy, there are websites out there that do this for you based on the activity, age, height and weight. After that, calculate how much protein you need (0.8-1.1 g/lb), then set aside 20-30% of your calories to come from fat and the rest from carbohydrates. Due to the variable of your weight and height I cannot recommend anything in this program.

With a higher amount of carbohydrates and fats allowed into your diet, you can have more energy to carry out strenuous strength training to gain strength and muscle mass and endurance.

Here's a simplified Table to show how you can easily plan out your daily calories intake during both cutting and muscle gain phase.

| RECOMMENDED MACRONUTRIENTS | PROTEIN | FAT | CARBOHYDRATE |
|---|---|---|---|
| RECOVERY | 1.1 – 1.3 grams per pound (2.3 – 2.0 g/ kg) of bodyweight | 20 – 30% of total calories per day | The remaining calories are filled with carbs |

# Recovery & Performance Enhancing Supplements

## Significance of Muscle Gaining Supplements

Generally, to build up muscle it is still better to achieve it via diet and exercise while supplementation should only be used for additive effects. Nonetheless, it should not be pushed aside as supplements are still generally used for health and building muscle. The Top 3 most used supplements are Creatine, Vitamin D and Omega – 3 Supplement from Fish Oil. You might wonder if Omega 3 fatty acids from flax/chia seeds should be considered as well, but the fact is flax/chia seeds do not provide sufficient supplement on its own. Flax/chia seeds are found in the form of Alpha-Linoleic Acid (ALA) which has to be converted by the body into a usable form and the ratio conversion is rather poor.

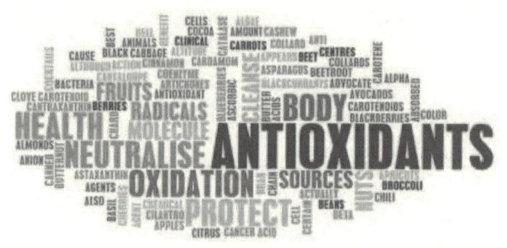

**Diet Plan Tip**: Foods are usually insufficient for anyone that is looking to gain muscles in the fastest manner, the best option is to take in the right supplements for your body needs.

## Top 3 Muscle Gaining Supplements

### Creatine / Creatine monohydrate

This is by far on the top of my performance supplement for muscle gains.

Creatine monohydrate is by far the most tried and true, most affordable, and effective of all the creatine variants. It is original, and many subsequent variants of creatine are either inferior or cost more without giving any additional benefit. So creatine monohydrate is the specific type that I recommend, instead of those packed with additional glucose or unnecessary 'proprietary blend' (Most likely another marketing gimmick to inflate the price).

We get most of our creatine from animal products, mostly in meat, and it is more abundant in raw meat. When the meat is cooked it degrades the creatine content, which is why it is difficult to get the performance-enhancing benefits without consuming this as a supplement.

To get creatine stores up to levels where they can benefit strength, power production, muscle fullness and ultimately your long-term ability to produce more muscle mass over time, I would recommend ingesting 0.018 g/lb of bodyweight per day (0.04 g/kg/ day). It will take a couple of weeks of ingesting this amount per day to reach supplemental creatine levels, but after that point, you can just maintain those levels by continuing to take the dose, like the topping of your gas tank.

And last but not least, it's important to note that for long-term consumption, timing doesn't matter. It doesn't need to be taken with carbs, it doesn't need to be loaded, it doesn't need to be taken pre-workout, and it doesn't need to be taken post-workout. All the benefits associated with creatine timing, whether it's taken with carbs, or if creatine is loaded in large amounts, are strictly related to the first couple weeks of consumption where the goal is to get to supplemental levels. It has nothing to do with long-term use and whether it takes you 5 days or 21 days to reach supplemental levels of creatine has a less than negligible effect on long-term gains. So, just take the daily dose I recommend and you'll be all set to reap its benefits.

## Vitamin D

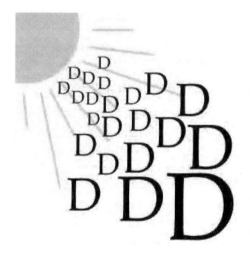

Vitamin D is primarily produced in our body as a result of direct contact with sunlight. Having insufficient levels of vitamin D in the body can compromise the immune system, which can be a disaster for someone who is training hard, dieting or attempting to perform any type of activity at a high level.

Vitamin D also affects our mood and hormonal level. Furthermore, it's frequently linked to depression and psychological breakdown (See how this could be important.)

Vitamin D deficiency rates are a lot higher than we think, and being deficient in Vitamin D can have negative impacts on muscular performance, immune function and hormonal status. Thus, it's a good idea to supplement accordingly if you don't get much direct sunlight, have dark skin or a combination thereof. A basic dosing recommendation would be to take anywhere from 1000-2000 IU/lb/day of vitamin D3 based on sunlight exposure. For those who find supplements that don't list the amount of Vitamin D3 in IU's, the equivalent dose in micrograms is 0.225 to 0.900 mcg/lbs/day (0.5 to 2 mcg/kg/day).

So if you work or train outdoors on a daily basis, you might not benefit from supplemental vitamin D3 at all. Perhaps taking 9 IU/lb (20 IU/kg) at most to be extra safe that you're getting enough would be a good idea. If you are someone on the opposite extreme end of the sunlight exposure spectrum, it might be more appropriate to take the full 36 IU/lb (80 IU/kg). So, you can regularly make sure to supplement the maximal effective dose throughout the winter, and in the summer, months stop taking Vitamin D supplements.

If possible, the absolute best route would be to get your blood work checked to see where your levels are and to see if you're deficient. Otherwise, just use your best estimate in the range provided based on lifestyle and exposure to sunlight.

**Supplement Facts**: Vitamin D deficiency is relatively common in athletes and is associated with muscle weakness and atrophy, specifically Type 2 muscle fiber atrophy. Skipping out on this vitamin is just as bad as skipping out on leg day.

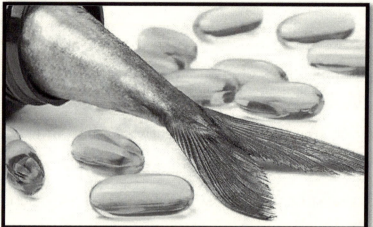

## Fish Oil

Of the essential fatty acids (EFA's), eicosapentaenoic acid (EPA) and docosahexaenoic acid (DHA), which typically come from fish oil supplementation, have been found to have a host of potential health benefits. If you don't eat fish or don't like taking fish oil, you can also get EPA and DHA from an algae supplement, which is what the fish eat that gives them the EPA and DHA that we are looking for.

When appropriately dosed, EFA's help with leptin signaling in the brain, reducing inflammation, enhancing mood and reducing disease factor risk. They can also aid in joint recovery and even as far as muscle development. 1 gram should suffice, however upwards to 6 grams has been taken for recovery.

## Rule of Thumb for a Good Diet

A good diet supposed to be simple and not to over-complicate things.

For tactical athletes, performance-based training, your priority is not food restrictions. Instead, you should be focusing on the number of calories you're going to take throughout the day.

For starters, I recommend tracking your daily calories intake to have a clear picture of how your diet looks like and how you can manipulate it afterward.

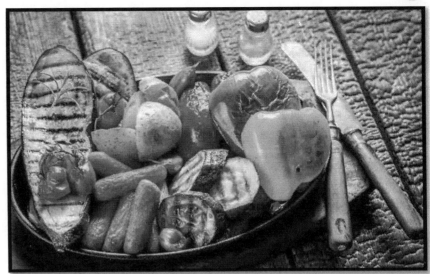

Next is to determine what are your macronutrients percentage and finally the essential micronutrients (which can be easily covered with supplements). Trust me, by becoming aware of your daily food intake, you will ultimately expedite recovery, giving you an edge by training harder and longer.

## Foods to avoid

Generally, you should be avoiding food that makes you feel 'bloated', 'sick' and 'low-energy'. This includes processed, highly-toxic (with chemicals), junk food and sugary foods. Sugar is the main factor that you should really look out for as it is present in foods particularly that aren't fresh, frozen or dried. Additionally, sauces such as pasta sauce, ketchup and chili sauce contain sugar as well. Moreover, fruit juices and fizzy drinks are things that you need to avoid as well.

## Supplements To Avoid

Supplements today are expensive! And if you're not careful, you'll end up burning a hole in your wallet with supplements that do not work.

There are a lot of people these days sold to the craze of muscle enhancing supplements that promise jaw-dropping muscle mass development. But honestly, do they even work? There are various supplements that would improve muscle growth but only a handful of them are actually scientifically proven to work if consumed in the recommended method. Supplements that do not offer any muscle growth are considered placebo pills and powders which is merely an implication to your mind that it affects your body.

## Testosterone Booster

They are supplements that increase testosterone levels in the blood, most of the compounds do boost testosterone levels, while others claim to do so, but in reality there is no actual proof that they do boost testosterone. It is recommended to cycle testosterone boosters as they do have side-effects that could be detrimental to your health if taken excessively. Like a negative feedback loop, in which estrogen levels increase in your body, these side effects generally are not excessive or common.

Studies show that testosterone booster can actually cause testicles atrophy and lower HPTA stimulation if used excessively or with prolonged usage.

Also, it is shown that some even developed "adrenal fatigue" due to the chemical compounds in boosters.

There are 3 prime examples of compounds that have been scientifically proven to not directly affect testosterone levels, however it can promote a healthy level, are ZMA, and D-aspartic acid and ecdysterone.

- ZMA is a combination of zinc, magnesium and vitamin B6 which is in the same line with Tribulus Terrestris. People who are deficient from zinc and magnesium would benefit their overall health but not by primarily increasing testosterone levels. It may have a secondary effect as ZMA could remove micronutrient deficiency that is suppressing testosterone production, which more common than you may think.

- D-aspartic acid can increase testosterone levels but the effects are short-lived and temporary, this can actually be used as a beneficial tool, used in cycles to promote overall recovery.

- Ecdysterone, one of my personal favorites. Ecdysterone (also known as ecdysteroids) can be found in plants, like spinach and cyanotis arachnodiea (has the highest content of ecdysterone.) This molecule has been found to have no toxicity or harmful side effects, yet can promote muscle growth and recovery at an incredible rate. Without affecting hormones. Sadly, most manufacturers either cut their supplements or have no detectable levels of this molecule. A recent study released by the Department of Molecular and Cellular Sports Medicine in May 2019 classified this as an anabolic substance.

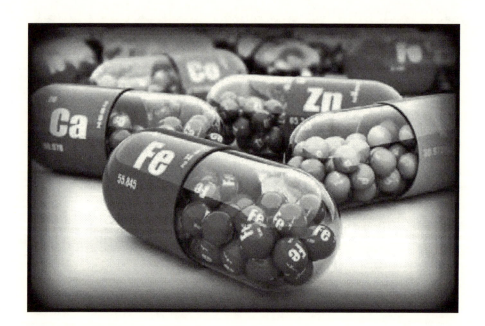

There are various scientific studies that have been conducted to determine if increasing testosterone levels could help with boosting muscle gains. The results pretty much show that no matter how high you increase your testosterone levels, it would not help boost muscle building compared to consuming proper diet meals and viable supplements.

**The key to building muscle is proper training and nutrition not reliance on supplements.**

## Protein Supplement Scams

We like protein powder. It's a quick, convenient and cost-effective way to hit our daily protein targets. Whey protein is not the cheapest, but it is popular due to the high BCAA content, particularly leucine, which is critical to the muscle-building process.

Now, with consumers becoming wiser there is a rising demand for products that claim to have been lab-tested, but this comes at a time of overall rising global demand (and thus prices). With consumers becoming sensitive to these price increases and a lack of general education about what they should be looking for on the packet, the incentives for companies to cut costs by cheating the system are all there, and many do. I'm talking about the rise of the phenomenon known as 'protein spiking'.

The way it works is this: some labs test for the total amino acid content rather than the amounts of the individual amino acids themselves. This means that protein companies can dump cheap amino acids into the mix (mainly glycine and taurine), skimping on the actual whey content, which is expensive, and yet still pass some quality tests. Here are some red flags to look out for when choosing a whey powder:

1. The cost per pound / kilo of claimed protein content is considerably cheaper than average. Whey is a commodity traded on the open market. You can be ripped off and pay way too much (You can even find places that sell 10x market price in luxury gyms!)

2. It has a proprietary blend (or doesn't list leucine content).

3. Leucine content, when listed, is lower than 2.7 g per 25 g of protein content (the BCAA content of whey is 25%, leucine should be 11%).

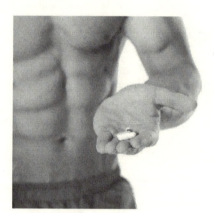

If your protein powder doesn't pass those checks, you're rolling the dice with the quality of what you're getting. Protein supplement consumption is entirely optional and is based on personal preference. You can still opt for dieting instead of taking in protein powders, which is the recommended way to get your protein in.

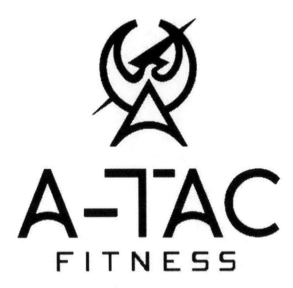

8-Week Beginner Fitness Program

# ARE YOU READY....

## LET'S BEGIN...

**THAT OTHERS MAY LIVE – FIRST THERE**

# WARM-UPS & DYNAMIC WARMUPS

We cannot stress the importance of making sure your muscles are loose and warmed up before starting your daily program. Do ANY of the following to make sure you got the juices flowing to take on the day right before starting your workout.

| <u>Warm-up (5-10min)</u> | <u>Dynamic Warmups</u> |
|---|---|
| Jump rope | 20x Leg Swings (Both Legs) |
| Light Jog | 20x Lunge and Twists |
| Cycling | 20x T-Pushups |
| Row (Easy & Light) | 20x Arm Circles (Both Arms) |
| Stair Climber (Easy) | 20x Leg Crossovers |

# WARM-UPS BEFORE GOING HEAVY (Weights)

Prior to weight lifting (Specifically Deadlifts & Bench press in this routine) do 3 warm-up sets of very light weight while slowly building up to that first real set in your workout. Rests between warm-up sets should be no more than 2 minutes long.

20 reps @ 15-20% of your maximum weight 7 reps @ 50% of Your maximum weight
6 reps @ 65-75% of your maximum weight

**\*Commence workout\***
**\*NOTE\*** Rests between the actual weight lifting routines (90%, 80%, 70%) should be about 3-4 minutes

# WEEK 1 OF 8

|           | CARDIO | PHYSICAL TRAINING | SWIM |
|-----------|--------|-------------------|------|
| **MONDAY** | o OFF | **Complete 3 Rounds for Time**<br>• Row machine- 500m in under 2 minutes (Row setting should be between 5-10)<br>• 2 Min rest<br>• 20 Kettle bell swings (25-35 lbs)<br>• 1 min rest<br>• 25 Flutter Kicks (4-Count)<br>• 1 min rest<br>• 20 pushups<br>• 1 min rest | o OFF |
| **TUESDAY** | • Warm up<br>• 1 mile run (70% effort)<br>**\*Note\*** If running on a treadmill be sure to do a 1% incline<br>• Stretch/ Cool down | o OFF | **Warm Up**<br>• 200m Freestyle (easy)<br>**Main Set**<br>• 6 x 100m Fin (75% effort)<br>**Cool Down**<br>• 100 meter swim (Any stroke) |
| **WEDNESDAY** | o OFF | **AS Many Reps As Possible (AMRAP) 13 Minutes**<br>*Try your hardest to maintain strict & proper form throughout the duration of the workout* NO SHORTCUTS!<br>o 10 pushups<br>o 10 sit-ups<br>o 5 pullups<br>o 10 air squats | **WARM UP:**<br>o 100m Freestyle, easy<br>**MAIN SET:**<br>o 4 x 50m Freestyle (fins), 95% effort, 1 min rest<br>o 1 x 300m Freestyle (fins), 70-80% effort, 3 min rest<br>**COOL DOWN:** 100m Freestyle (fins), easy |
| **THURSDAY** | • Warm up<br>• 1-Mile run (7:30- min Pace)<br>**\*Note\*** If running on a treadmill be sure to do a 1% incline<br>• Cool Down / Stretch | **Complete 3 Rounds for Time**<br>• 12 Jumping Pull ups<br>• 12 body weight rows<br>• 6 chin ups<br>• 10 leg lifts<br>• 30 second plank (left Side)<br>• 30 second plank (Right side)<br>• 30 second plank (Center)<br>• 15 wide pushups<br>• 15 Kettle Bell swings (25-35 lbs) | o OFF |
| **FRIDAY** | o OFF | **Complete 1 Round of Each**<br>o 6x DEAD LIFTS (90% OF MAX)<br>o 8x DEAD LIFTS (80% OF MAX)<br>o 10x DEAD LIFTS (70% OF MAX)<br>o 6x BENCH PRESS OR DB PRESS (90% OF MAX)<br>o 8x BENCH PRESS OR DB PRESS (80% OF MAX)<br>o 10x BENCH PRESS OR DB PRESS (70% OF MAX)<br>**Complete 3 Rounds of Each**<br>o 15 CHIN UPS<br>o 15 HANGING LEG RAISES<br>o 20 BICYCLES (4 count)<br>o 25 PUSHUPS<br>o 20 LEG RAISES<br>o 10 DIPS | **WARM UP:**<br>o 100m Freestyle, easy<br>**MAIN SET:**<br>o 6 x 100m Freestyle (fins), 95% effort, 1 min rest<br>o 1 x 500m Freestyle (No fins), 70-80% effort, 3 min rest<br>**COOL DOWN:** 150m Freestyle, easy |
| **SATURDAY** | o REST<br>o STRETCH/ FOAM ROLL | o REST<br>o STRETCH/ FOAM ROLL | o REST<br>o STRETCH/ FOAM ROLL |
| **SUNDAY** | o REST<br>o STRETCH/ FOAM ROLL | o REST<br>o STRETCH/ FOAM ROLL | o REST<br>o STRETCH/ FOAM ROLL |

# WEEK 2 OF 8

| | CARDIO | PHYSICAL TRAINING | SWIM |
|---|---|---|---|
| **MONDAY** | o Dynamic Warm-up<br>o 400M INTERVALS: 90 sec on/90 sec off (400M =1 Lap around the track) in 90 sec Rest 90 sec. Repeat. Run for a total of 1 Mile (4 laps)<br>*Note* If running on a treadmill be sure to do a 1% incline<br>o Cool Down / Stretch | **Complete 3 rounds**<br>o 35 PUSHUPS<br>o 10 DIAMOND PUSHUPS<br>o 15 MODIFIED V-SITS (4 count)<br>o 15 CLAPPING PUSHUPS<br>o 30 FLUTTER KICKS (4 count)<br>o 20 DECLINE PUSHUPS<br>o 20 WIDE PUSHUPS<br>o 30 SECOND SIDE PLANKS (each side)<br>o 6 BODYWEIGHT TRICEP EXTENSION (STRAIGHT BAR) | o OFF |
| **TUESDAY** | o OFF | **Complete 3 Rounds for Time**<br>o 15 MOUNTAIN CLIMBERS (4 COUNT)<br>o 10 GLUTE HAM RAISE<br>o 30 FLUTTER KICKS (4 COUNT)<br>o 10 DIPS<br>o 10 PULL-UPS<br>o 40 SECOND SIDE PLANKS (each side)<br>o 10 CLOSE GRIP PULL UPS<br>o 12 DIVE BOMBERS<br>o 10 WIDE GRIP PULLUPS<br>o 10 BODY WEIGHT ROWS (OVER HAND)<br>o 10 BODY WEIGHT ROWS (UNDERHAND) | **WARM UP:**<br>o 200m Freestyle, easy (fins)<br>**MAIN SET:**<br>o 3 x 100m Lead arm- Trail arm (fins), 95% effort, 30 sec rest<br>o 1 x 500m Lead arm- Trail arm (fins), 70-80% effort, 2 min rest<br>**COOL DOWN:** 100m Lead arm- Trail arm OR Freestyle, easy |
| **WEDNESDAY** | • Dynamic Warm-up<br>• 1.25 Mile Max Effort<br>*Note* If running on a treadmill be sure to do a 1% incline<br>• Cool Down / Stretch | o OFF | **WARM UP:**<br>o 200m Freestyle, easy<br>**MAIN SET:**<br>o 6 x 100m Lead arm- Trail arm (fins), 95% effort, 1 min rest<br>o 600 x m Lead arm- Trail arm (fins), 70-80% effort, 3 min rest<br>o 3 x 100m Lead arm- Trail arm , 70% effort, 30 sec rest<br>**COOL DOWN:** 100m Lead arm- Trail arm, easy |
| **THURSDAY** | o OFF | **MAN MAKERS**<br>Start with 10 reps, then 9, then 8…all the way down to one<br>15-25lb Dumbbells<br>10-9-8-7-6- 5-4-3-2-1 | o OFF |
| **FRIDAY** | o OFF | **COMPLETE 4 ROUNDS FOR TIME**<br>o 15 IRON MIKES (4 COUNT)<br>o 25 PUSH UPS<br>o 25 AIR SQUATS<br>o 30 FLUTTER KICKS (4 COUNT)<br>o 15 GOBLET SQUATS<br>o 15 LEG LIFTS<br>o 10 BURPEES<br>o 20 SIT UPS | **WARM UP:**<br>o 200m Freestyle<br>o 200m Combat Side Stroke, easy (fins)<br>**MAIN SET:**<br>o 4 x 100m Lead arm- Trail arm (fins), 95% effort, 1 min rest<br>o 1 x 700m Lead arm- Trail arm (fins), 70-80% effort, 30 sec rest<br>**COOL DOWN:** 100m Lead arm- Trail arm, easy |
| **SATURDAY** | o REST<br>o STRETCH/ FOAM ROLL | o REST<br>o STRETCH/ FOAM ROLL | o REST<br>o STRETCH/ FOAM ROLL |
| **SUNDAY** | o REST<br>o STRETCH/ FOAM ROLL | o REST<br>o STRETCH/ FOAM ROLL | o REST<br>o STRETCH/ FOAM ROLL |

# WEEK 3 OF 8

|  | CARDIO | PHYSICAL TRAINING | SWIM |
|---|---|---|---|
| **MONDAY** | o OFF | **Complete 3 Rounds for Time**<br>• Dynamic Warm Up<br>• Row machine- 500m in under 2 minutes (Row setting should be between 5-10)<br>• 2 Min rest<br>• 25 Kettle bell swings (25-35 lbs)<br>• 1 min rest<br>• 30 Flutter Kicks (4-Count)<br>• 1 min rest<br>• 25 pushups<br>• 1 min rest | o OFF |
| **TUESDAY** | o OFF | **Complete 1 set of ALL workouts below**<br>o DYNAMIC WARM UP<br>o 6x DEAD LIFTS (90% OF MAX)<br>o 8x DEAD LIFTS (80% OF MAX)<br>o 10x DEAD LIFTS (70% OF MAX)<br>o 6x BENCH PRESS OR DB PRESS (90% OF MAX)<br>o 8x BENCH PRESS OR DB PRESS (80% OF MAX)<br>o 10x BENCH PRESS OR DB PRESS (70% OF MAX)<br>**Complete 3 sets of Each**<br>o 15x MODIFIED V SITS<br>o LEFT PLANK (40 SEC)<br>o RIGHT PLANK (40 SEC)<br>o CENTER PLANK (40 SEC) | **WARM UP:**<br>o 200m Freestyle<br>**MAIN SET:**<br>o 3 x 100m Lead arm- Trail arm (fins), 95% effort, 30 sec rest<br>o 1 x 600m Lead arm- Trail arm, 70-80% effort, 2 min rest<br>**COOL DOWN:** 100m Lead arm- Trail arm (fins), easy |
| **WEDNESDAY** | o Dynamic Warm-up<br>o 400M INTERVALS: 90 sec on/90 sec off (400M =1 Lap around the track) in 90 sec. Rest 90 sec. Repeat. Run for a total of 1.25 Miles (5 laps)<br>*Note* If running on a treadmill be sure to do a 1% incline<br>o Cool Down / Stretch | o OFF | **WARM UP:**<br>o 200m Freestyle<br>**MAIN SET:**<br>o 4 x 100m Lead arm- Trail arm (fins), 95% effort, 1 min rest<br>o 1 x 600m Combat Side Stroke (fins), 70-80% effort, 30 sec rest<br>**COOL DOWN:** 100m Lead arm- Trail arm (fins), easy |
| **THURSDAY** | o OFF | **Complete 5 Rounds**<br>o DYNAMIC WARM UP<br>o 10x 8 COUNT BODY BUILDERS<br>o 2 MIN REST<br>o 400M RUN IN 90 SEC<br>o 2 MIN REST<br>o REPEAT FOR 5 ROUNDS | o OFF |
| **FRIDAY** | o Dynamic Warm-up<br>o 1.5 Mile Run<br>• Moderate Effort<br>*Note* If running on a treadmill be sure to do a 1% incline<br>o Cool Down / Stretch | **AMRAP (AS MANY REPS AS POSSIBLE) 20 MIN**<br>o 5 PULL UPS<br>o 12 PUSH UPS<br>o 12 SIT UPS<br>o 15 AIR SQUATS | **MAIN SET:**<br>o 1 x 500m Freestyle, EASY (no fins), 60-70% effort (Recovery Swim)<br>o **COOL DOWN:** 150m Freestyle, easy |
| **SATURDAY** | o REST<br>o STRETCH/ FOAM ROLL | o REST<br>o STRETCH/ FOAM ROLL | o REST<br>o STRETCH/ FOAM ROLL |
| **SUNDAY** | o REST<br>o STRETCH/ FOAM ROLL | o REST<br>o STRETCH/ FOAM ROLL | o REST<br>o STRETCH/ FOAM ROLL |

# WEEK 4 OF 8

| | CARDIO | PHYSICAL TRAINING | SWIM |
|---|---|---|---|
| **MONDAY** | - Dynamic Warm-up<br>- 2 Mile Run<br>  - Max Effort<br>*Note* If running on a treadmill be sure to do a 1% incline<br>Cool Down / Stretch | **Complete 3 Rounds (GRIP STRENGTH)**<br>- 45 SEC DEADHANG FROM PULLUP BAR<br>- 12 DIPS<br>- 10 HANGING KNEES TO ELBOWS<br>- 10 SHOULDER SHRUGS (25-45LBS EACH ARM)<br>- 12 BODYWEIGHT ROWS (UNDERHAND)<br>- 12 BODY WEIGHT ROWS (OVERHAND)<br>- 10x BENTOVER DUMBBELL ROWS (70% MAX)<br>- 10x SEATED ROWS (70% MAX)<br>- PULL UPS UNTIL FAILURE | - OFF |
| **TUESDAY** | - OFF | **MURPH WORKOUT FOR TIME**<br>- 1 MILE (AIM FOR 7 MIN MILE)<br>- 100 PULLUPS<br>- 200 PUSHUPS<br>- 300 AIR SQUATS<br>- 1 MILE (AIM FOR 7 MIN MILE) | - OFF |
| **WEDNESDAY** | - Dynamic Warm-up<br>- 2 Mile Run<br>  - Moderate Effort (70%)<br>*Note* If running on a treadmill be sure to do a 1% incline<br>- Cool Down / Stretch | - OFF | **WARM UP:**<br>- 250m Freestyle, easy<br>**MAIN SET:**<br>- 3 x 100m Lead arm- Trail arm (fins), 95% effort, 1 min rest<br>- 1 x 700m Lead arm- Trail arm (fins), 70 effort, 3 min rest<br>- 3x100m Lead arm- Trail arm (fins), 75% effort, 20 sec rest<br>**COOL DOWN:** 200m Lead arm- Trail arm, easy |
| **THURSDAY** | - OFF | **Complete 3 Rounds for Time**<br>- 30 PUSHUPS<br>- 25 SHOULDER CIRCLES AKA SUN GODS (4 count)<br>- 30 BICYCLES (4 count)<br>- 30 DIAMOND PUSHUPS<br>- 12 DIVE BOMBERS<br>- 30 SIT UPS<br>- 15 SHOULDER Pushups<br>- 30 WIDE PUSHUPS<br>- 1 MINUTE PLANK (LEFT, RIGHT & CENTER)<br>- 35 FLUTTER KICKS (4 COUNT)<br>- 10 BODY WEIGHT TRICEP EXTENSION (STRAIGHT BAR) | - OFF |
| **FRIDAY** | - OFF | **3 Rounds**<br>- 25 JUMPING AIR SQUATS<br>- 15 IRON MIKES (4 COUNT)<br>- ALTERNATING LUNGES (10ea LEG)<br>- 10 GOBLET SQUATS (25-45LBS)<br>- 12 JUMPING PULL UPS<br>- 10 PLYO SPLIT SQUAT (10ea LEG)<br>- 30 SIT UPS<br>- 10 V-UPS<br>- SINGLE LEG BOSU BALL BALANCE (30 SEC each LEG) | **WARM UP:**<br>- 250m Freestyle, easy<br>**MAIN SET:**<br>- 4 x 100m Combat Side stroke- (fins), 95% effort, 90 sec rest<br>- 1 x 600m Combat Side Stroke (fins), 70 effort, 2 min rest<br>**COOL DOWN:** 200m Freestyle (fins), easy |
| **SATURDAY** | - REST<br>- STRETCH/ FOAM ROLL | - REST<br>- STRETCH/ FOAM ROLL | - REST<br>- STRETCH/ FOAM ROLL |
| **SUNDAY** | - REST<br>- STRETCH/ FOAM ROLL | - REST<br>- STRETCH/ FOAM ROLL | - REST<br>- STRETCH/ FOAM ROLL |

# WEEK 5 OF 8

|  | CARDIO | PHYSICAL TRAINING | SWIM |
|---|---|---|---|
| **MONDAY** | - Dynamic Warm-up<br>- 1.5 Mile Run<br>  - Max Effort<br><br>*Note* If running on a treadmill be sure to do a 1% incline<br><br>- Cool Down / Stretch | **Complete 1 Rounds**<br>- PULL UPS (STRICT FORM) AS MANY AS POSSIBLE- 2 MIN<br>- PUSH UPS (STRICT FORM) AS MANY AS POSSIBLE- 2 MIN<br>- SIT UPS (STRICT FORM) AS MANY AS POSSIBLE- 2 MIN<br>- RECORD REPS | **MAIN SET:**<br>- 500M FREE STYLE (NO FINS)<br>- MAX EFFORT<br>- RECORD TIME |
| **TUESDAY** | - OFF | **MAN MAKERS**<br><br>Start with 10 reps, then 9, then 8…all the way down to one<br><br>15-25lb Dumbbells<br><br>10-9-8-7-6- 5-4-3-2-1 | **WARM UP:**<br>- Freestyle 300M, easy<br>**MAIN SET:**<br>- 3 x 200m Lead arm- Trail arm , 85% effort, 2 min rest<br>- 2 x 500m Lead arm- Trail arm (fins), 70 effort, 3 min rest<br>**COOL DOWN:** 100m Lead arm- Trail arm (fins), easy<br>**TOTAL: 2000m** |
| **WEDNESDAY** | - OFF | **Complete 3 Rounds for Time**<br>- 30 DIAMOND PUSHUPS<br>- 35 PUSHUPS<br>- 15 RUSSIAN TWISTS (4 count)<br>- 15 DIPS<br>- 10 LUNGES (each leg) (overhead plate carry preferred 25-45lb)<br>- 20 LEG RAISES<br>- 10 DIVE BOMBERS<br>- 30 WIDE PUSHUPS<br>- 30 SECOND L-SITS<br>- 12 BODYWEIGHT TRICEPS EXTENSIONS<br>- 25 CALF RAISES (each leg)<br>- 35 BICYCLES (4 count) | **WARM UP:**<br>- Freestyle 300m, easy<br>**MAIN SET:**<br>- 2 x 500m Lead arm- Trail arm (fins), 85% effort, 30 sec rest<br>**COOL DOWN:** 100m Lead arm- Trail arm , easy |
| **THURSDAY** | - Dynamic Warm-up<br>- Run 1 mile at 7:00 min pace<br>- Rest for 4 min<br>- Run 2 miles at 7:45 min pace, rest 5 min<br>- Run 1 mile at 7:00 min pace<br>*Note* If running on a treadmill be sure to do a 1% incline<br><br>- Cool Down / Stretch | - OFF | - OFF |
| **FRIDAY** | - OFF | **Complete 3 Rounds for Time**<br>- 10 PULL UPS<br>- 10 CHIN UPS<br>- 30 BICYCLES (4 count)<br>- 35 FLUTTER KICKS (4 COUNT)<br>- 15 BACK EXTENSIONS<br>- 20 LEG LIFTS<br>- 15 BODYWEIGHT ROWS (OVER HAND)<br>- 15 SHOULDER Pushups<br>- 15 BODY WEIGHT ROWS (UNDER HAND)<br>- 10 HANGING KNEES TO BAR<br>- 8 WIDE PULL UPS<br>- 45 SECOND PLANK (LEFT, RIGHT & CENTER) | **WARM UP:**<br>- 300m Combat Side Stroke (w/ or without fins)<br>- 100m Lead arm- Trail arm, easy (fins)<br>**MAIN SET:**<br>- 3 x 100m Lead arm- Trail arm (fins), 95% effort, 2 min rest<br>- 3 x 200m Lead arm- Trail arm (fins), 85% effort, 2 min rest<br>- 1 x 500m Lead arm- Trail arm , 70% effort, 4 min rest<br>**COOL DOWN:** 100m Lead arm- Trail arm (fins), easy |
| **SATURDAY** | - REST<br>- STRETCH/ FOAM ROLL | - REST<br>- STRETCH/ FOAM ROLL | - REST<br>- STRETCH/ FOAM ROLL |
| **SUNDAY** | - REST<br>- STRETCH/ FOAM ROLL | - REST<br>- STRETCH/ FOAM ROLL | - REST<br>- STRETCH/ FOAM ROLL |

# WEEK 6 OF 8

| | CARDIO | PHYSICAL TRAINING | SWIM |
|---|---|---|---|
| **MONDAY** | o OFF | **Complete 4 Rounds for Time**<br>o Row machine- 500m in under 2 minutes (Row setting should be between 5-10)<br>o 2 Min rest<br>o 25 Kettle bell swings (25-35 lbs)<br>o 1 min rest<br>o 40 Flutter Kicks (4-Count)<br>o 1 min rest<br>o 35 pushups<br>o 1 min rest | OFF |
| **TUESDAY** | o Dynamic Warm-up<br>o 2.5 Mile Run (Aim for 7 min per mile)<br>• Moderate Effort (70%)<br>***Note*** If running on a treadmill be sure to do a 1% incline<br>o Cool Down / Stretch | OFF | **WARM UP:**<br>o 300m Freestyle<br>**MAIN SET:**<br>o 3 x 100m Combat side stroke (fins), 95% effort, 3 min rest<br>o 2 x 200m Lead arm- Trail arm (fins), 85% effort, 2 min rest<br>o 1 x 500m Lead arm- Trail arm (fins), 70% effort, 1 min rest<br>**COOL DOWN:** 100m Lead arm- Trail arm (fins), easy |
| **WEDNESDAY** | o OFF | **Complete 6 Rounds**<br>o DYNAMIC WARM UP<br>o 15x 8 COUNT BODY BUILDERS<br>o 2 MIN REST<br>o 400M RUN IN 90 SEC<br>o 2 MIN REST<br>o REPEAT FOR 6 ROUNDS | **WARM UP:**<br>o 300m Freestyle, easy<br>**MAIN SET:**<br>o 3 x 100m Lead arm- Trail arm, (fins) 95% effort, 3 min rest<br>o 3 x 200m Lead arm- Trail arm (fins), 85% effort, 3 min rest<br>o 2 x 500m Lead arm- Trail arm (fins), 70-80% effort, 2 min rest<br>**COOL DOWN:** 200m Combat Side Stroke, easy |
| **THURSDAY** | o Dynamic Warm-up<br>o Run 2.5 miles- 100m on/ 100m off for a total of 2.5 miles<br>***Note*** If running on a treadmill be sure to do a 1% incline<br>o Cool Down / Stretch | o OFF | o OFF |
| **FRIDAY** | o OFF | **Complete 1 set of ALL workouts below**<br>o DYNAMIC WARM UP<br>o 6x DEAD LIFTS (90% OF MAX)<br>o 8x DEAD LIFTS (80% OF MAX)<br>o 10x DEAD LIFTS (70% OF MAX)<br>o 6x BENCH PRESS OR DB PRESS (90% OF MAX)<br>o 8x BENCH PRESS OR DB PRESS (80% OF MAX)<br>o 10x BENCH PRESS OR DB PRESS (70% OF MAX)<br>**Complete 3 sets of Each**<br>o 15x MODIFIED V SITS (4 count)<br>o LEFT PLANK (45 SEC)<br>o RIGHT PLANK (45 SEC)<br>o CENTER PLANK (45 SEC) | **WARM UP:**<br>o Freestyle 300m, easy<br>**MAIN SET:**<br>o 1 x 100m Lead arm- Trail arm (fins), 70% effort, 3 min rest<br>o 1 x 1000m Lead arm- Trail arm (fins), 70% effort, 30 sec rest<br>**COOL DOWN:** 200m Combat Side Stroke, easy |
| **SATURDAY** | o REST<br>o STRETCH/ FOAM ROLL | o REST<br>o STRETCH/ FOAM ROLL | o REST<br>o STRETCH/ FOAM ROLL |
| **SUNDAY** | o REST<br>o STRETCH/ FOAM ROLL | o REST<br>o STRETCH/ FOAM ROLL | o REST<br>o STRETCH/ FOAM ROLL |

# WEEK 7 OF 8

|  | CARDIO | PHYSICAL TRAINING | SWIM |
|---|---|---|---|
| **MONDAY** | - Dynamic Warm-up<br>- 400M INTERVALS: 90 sec on/90 sec off (400M =1 Lap around the track) in 90 sec. Rest 90 sec. Repeat. Run for a total of 1.5 Miles (6 laps)<br>- *Note* If running on a treadmill be sure to do a 1% incline<br>- Cool Down / Stretch | **AS Many Reps As Possible (AMRAP) 20 Minutes**<br>*Try your hardest to maintain strict & proper form throughout the duration of the workout* NO SHORTCUTS!<br>- 12 pushups<br>- 15 sit-ups<br>- 6 pullups<br>- 12 air squats | - OFF |
| **TUESDAY** | - OFF | **Complete 3 Rounds**<br>- 15 BURPEES<br>- 15 8-COUNT BODYBUILDERS<br>- 40 FLUTTER KICKS (4 count)<br>- 30 AIR SQUATS<br>- PUSH UP POSITION HOLD FOR 1 MIN (try not to dip or arch your back as much as possible)<br>- 50 SIT UPS<br>- SINGLE LEG BOSU BALL BALANCE (45 SEC each LEG)<br>- 20 RUSSIAN TWISTS (4 count)<br>- 25 CALF RAISES (each leg)<br>- 25 KETTLE BELL SWINGS (25-50LB)<br>- 15 GLUTE HAM RAISES | **WARM UP:**<br>- 300m Freestyle<br>- 200m Combat Side Stroke, easy (fins)<br>**MAIN SET:**<br>- 3 x 100m Lead arm- Trail arm (fins), 95% effort, 1 min rest<br>- 1 x 800m Lead arm- Trail arm (fins), 70-80% effort, 2 min rest<br>**COOL DOWN:** 100 m Lead arm- Trail arm , easy |
| **WEDNESDAY** | - Dynamic Warm-up<br>- 2.75 Mile Run<br>  - Moderate Effort (70%)<br>*Note* If running on a treadmill be sure to do a 1% incline<br>- Cool Down / Stretch | - OFF | **WARM UP:**<br>- 300m Freestyle<br>- 100m Lead arm- Trail arm, easy (fins)<br>**MAIN SET:**<br>- 1 x 1000m Lead arm- Trail arm , 70-80% effort, 1 min rest<br>**COOL DOWN:** 100 m Lead arm- Trail arm (fins), easy |
| **THURSDAY** | - OFF | **Complete 3 rounds (Grip Strength)**<br>- 1 MIN DEADHANG FROM PULLUP BAR<br>- 15 DIPS<br>- 12 HANGING KNEES TO ELBOWS<br>- 10 SHOULDER SHRUGS (25-45LBS EACH ARM)<br>- 15 BODYWEIGHT ROWS (UNDERHAND)<br>- 15 BODY WEIGHT ROWS (OVERHAND)<br>- 10x BENTOVER DUMBBELL ROWS (70% MAX)<br>- 10x SEATED ROWS (70% MAX)<br>- PULL UPS UNTIL FAILURE | OFF |
| **FRIDAY** | - Dynamic Warm-up<br>- Run 2.75 miles- 100m on/ 100m off for a total of 2.75 miles (7 LAPS)<br>*Note* If running on a treadmill be sure to do a 1% incline<br>- Cool Down / Stretch | - OFF | **WARM UP:**<br>- 200m Freestyle<br>**MAIN SET:**<br>- 1 x 600m free style, 70% effort, easy<br>**COOL DOWN:**<br>- 200m Combat Side Stroke, easy (NO fins) |
| **SATURDAY** | - REST<br>- STRETCH/ FOAM ROLL | - REST<br>- STRETCH/ FOAM ROLL | - REST<br>- STRETCH/ FOAM ROLL |
| **SUNDAY** | - REST<br>- STRETCH/ FOAM ROLL | - REST<br>- STRETCH/ FOAM ROLL | - REST<br>- STRETCH/ FOAM ROLL |

# WEEK 8 OF 8

|  | **CARDIO** | **PHYSICAL TRAINING** | **SWIM** |
|---|---|---|---|
| **MONDAY** | - Dynamic Warm-up<br>- Timed 3 Mile<br>  - Max Effort<br><br>*Note* If running on a treadmill be sure to do a 1% incline<br><br>- Cool Down / Stretch | **Complete 3 Rounds for Time**<br>- 30 BURPEES<br>- 30 8-COUNT BODY BUILDERS<br>- 35 BICYCLES (4 COUNT)<br>- 50 FLUTTER KICKS (4 COUNT)<br>- 25 KETTLE BELL SWINGS (25-50LB)<br>- 20 OVERHEAD PLATE SIT UPS (25LB)<br>- 45 PUSHUPS | - OFF |
| **TUESDAY** | - OFF | **Complete 5 Rounds for Time**<br>- Row machine- 500m in under 2 minutes (Row setting should be between 5-10)<br>- 2 Min rest<br>- 30 Kettle bell swings (25-50 lbs)<br>- 1 min rest<br>- 50 Flutter Kicks (4-Count)<br>- 1 min rest<br>- 45 pushups<br>- 1 min rest | **WARM UP:**<br>- 400m Freestyle<br>- 200m Lead arm- Trail arm, easy<br>**MAIN SET:**<br>- 1 x 1200m Lead arm- Trail arm (fins), 70-80% effort<br>**COOL DOWN:** 100m Combat side stroke, easy |
| **WEDNESDAY** | - Dynamic Warm-up<br>- 400M INTERVALS: 90 sec on/90 sec off (400M =1 Lap around the track) in 90 sec. Rest 90 sec. Repeat. Run for a total of 2 Miles (8 laps)<br><br>*Note* If running on a treadmill be sure to do a 1% incline<br><br>- Cool Down / Stretch | - OFF | **WARM UP:**<br>- 400m Freestyle<br>- 300m Lead arm- Trail arm, easy<br>**MAIN SET:**<br>- 2 x 200m Lead arm- Trail arm (fins), 85% effort, 2 min rest<br>- 3 x 600m Lead arm- Trail arm (fins), 70% effort, 2 min rest<br>**COOL DOWN:** 200m Combat Side stroke, easy |
| **THURSDAY** | - OFF | **3 Rounds**<br>- 30 JUMPING AIR SQUATS<br>- 20 IRON MIKES (4 COUNT)<br>- ALTERNATING LUNGES (10ea LEG)<br>- 20 GOBLET SQUATS (25-45LBS)<br>- 15 JUMPING PULL UPS<br>- 10 PLYO SPLIT SQUAT (10ea LEG)<br>- 50 SIT UPS<br>- 10 V-UPS<br>- SINGLE LEG BOSU BALL BALANCE (30 SEC each LEG)<br>- PUSHUPS UNTIL FAILURE<br>- PULL UPS UNTIL FAILURE | - OFF |
| **FRIDAY** | - Dynamic Warm-up<br>- 3 Mile Run<br>  - Moderate to Max Effort<br><br>*Note* If running on a treadmill be sure to do a 1% incline<br><br>- Cool Down / Stretch | **Complete 1 set of ALL workouts below**<br>- DYNAMIC WARM UP<br>- 6x DEAD LIFTS (90% OF MAX)<br>- 8x DEAD LIFTS (80% OF MAX)<br>- 10x DEAD LIFTS (70% OF MAX)<br>- 6x BENCH PRESS OR DB PRESS (90% OF MAX)<br>- 8x BENCH PRESS OR DB PRESS (80% OF MAX)<br>- 10x BENCH PRESS OR DB PRESS (70% OF MAX)<br>**Complete 3 sets of Each**<br>- 20x MODIFIED V SITS (4 count)<br>- LEFT PLANK (45 SEC)<br>- RIGHT PLANK (45 SEC)<br>- CENTER PLANK (45 SEC) | - OFF |
| **SATURDAY** | - REST<br>- STRETCH/ FOAM ROLL | - REST<br>- STRETCH/ FOAM ROLL | - REST<br>- STRETCH/ FOAM ROLL |
| **SUNDAY** | - REST<br>- STRETCH/ FOAM ROLL | - REST<br>- STRETCH/ FOAM ROLL | - REST<br>- STRETCH/ FOAM ROLL |

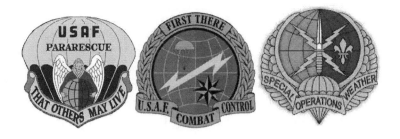

# Pararescue/Combat Control/Special Operations Weather Team (PJ/CCT/SOWT) Fitness Preparation Program

# INTRODUCTION

This program is intended to prepare candidates for the INTENSE physical demands of the PJ/CCT/SOWT training pipelines. It is a 26-week program created for candidates to attain a high state of physical readiness prior to entering active duty.

**Do not attempt this workout without first being cleared by a physician**. Many of these exercises are strenuous and may cause injury if you have existing medical conditions or you are not accustomed to exercising on a regular basis.

After being cleared by your physician, do not progress to a new week workout without having successfully completing the previous week workout. You may be putting yourself at risk of injury if you advance to the next workout without completing the previous workouts.

Once you get started on the program, pay close attention to how each exercise should be performed. Proper form **MUST** be maintained throughout all exercise movements. When done properly you will maximize your results and minimize injury risk. If you experience shortness of breath, dizziness, or chest pain during exercise you should discontinue the exercise and seek medical attention.

A few things to remember:

1. **NEVER** swim alone.
2. **ALWAYS** have a swim buddy.
3. If you cannot find a swim buddy, at least, swim in a pool with a lifeguard on duty.
4. If at any point in the program something doesn't feel right or you think you may have injured yourself, consult a physician.
5. **Always** complete a dynamic warm-up prior to exercise routine.


For further information or guidance, contact your nearest Special Operations Recruiting Liaison.

*THAT OTHERS MAY LIVE...*

# PHASE 1 WORKOUT
## WEEK 1 OF 11

| | CARDIO | PHYSICAL TRAINING | SWIM |
|---|---|---|---|
| **MONDAY** | - Dynamic Warm-up<br>- Timed Run<br>  - 30-40 min<br>  - Moderate Effort<br>- Cool Down / Stretch | **Complete 3 Rounds**<br>- 20 PUSH UPS<br>- 30 AIR SQUATS<br>- 20 SIT UPS<br>- 15 WIDE GRIP PUSHUPS<br>- 10 LUNGES (each leg)<br>- 20 FLUTTER KICKS (4 count)<br>- 10 DIAMOND PUSHUPS<br>- 10 GLUTE BRIDGES<br>- 30 SECOND PLANK | - OFF |
| **TUESDAY** | - OFF | **Complete 3 Rounds**<br>- 6 PULL UPS<br>- SINGLE LEG ROMANIAN DEADLIFT (no weight)<br>- 20 BICYCLES (4 count)<br>- 12 BODYWEIGHT ROWS<br>- 15 METER CRABWALK<br>- 20 SIT UPS<br>- 10 SUPERMANS<br>- 5 GLUTE HAM RAISE (Nordic Hamstring Curl)<br>- 30 SECOND SIDE PLANKS (each side) | **WARM UP:**<br>- 300m kick, bottom arm out straight (no fins)<br>- 100m Freestyle, easy<br>**MAIN SET:**<br>- 4 x 50m Freestyle (No fins), 95% effort, 30 sec rest<br>- 1 x 500m Freestyle (fins), 70-80% effort, 2 min rest<br>**COOL DOWN:** 200m Freestylee, easy<br>**TOTAL:** 1300m |
| **WEDNESDAY** | - Dynamic Warm-up<br>- Interval Workout 1<br>  - Reference Interval Generator for times<br>- Cool Down / Stretch | - OFF | **WARM UP:**<br>- 300m kick, bottom arm out straight (no fins)<br>- 200m Freestyle, easy<br>**MAIN SET:**<br>- 4 x 50m Freestyle (fins), 95% effort, 30 sec rest<br>- 2 x 500m Freestyle (No fins), 70-80% effort, 4 min rest<br>**COOL DOWN:** 100m Freestyle, easy<br>**TOTAL:** 1800m |
| **THURSDAY** | - OFF | **Complete as Fast as Possible**<br>- 30 BURPEES<br>- 30 SIT UPS<br>- 20 BURPEES<br>- 20 SIT UPS<br>- 10 BURPEES<br>- 10 SIT UPS | - OFF |
| **FRIDAY** | - Dynamic Warm-up<br>- Timed 1-mile<br>  - Max Effort<br>- Cool Down / Stretch | **Complete 3 Rounds**<br>- 6 CHIN UPS<br>- 10 DIAMOND PUSHUPS<br>- 15 MODIFIED V-SIT<br>- 12 UNDERHAND BODYWEIGHT ROWS<br>- 10 DIPS<br>- 45 SECOND PLANK<br>- 15 SECOND CHIN UP HOLD<br>- 10 SPHINX PUSHUPS<br>- 10 RUSSIAN TWISTS (4 count) | - OFF |
| **SATURDAY** | OFF | **Complete 3 Rounds**<br>- 15 SHOULDER CIRCLES (4 count; ea direction)<br>- 15 CALF RAISES<br>- 20 SIT UPS<br>- 20 METER INCHWORMS<br>- 1 MINUTE SQUAT HOLD<br>- 10 PLANK REACHES<br>- 6 DIVE BOMBER PUSHUPS<br>- 10 SQUAT JUMPS<br>- 20 LEG RAISES | **WARM UP:**<br>- 200m kick, bottom arm out straight (no fins)<br>- 100m Freestyle, easy<br>**MAIN SET:**<br>- 4 x 50m Freestyle (No fins), 95% effort, 30 sec rest<br>- 2 x 300m Freestyle (fins), 70-80% effort, 1 min rest<br>**COOL DOWN:** 200m Freestyle, easy<br>**TOTAL:** 1300m |
| **SUNDAY** | - OFF | - OFF | - OFF |

# PHASE 1 WORKOUT
## WEEK 2 OF 11

|  | CARDIO | PHYSICAL TRAINING | SWIM |
|---|---|---|---|
| **MONDAY** | - Dynamic Warm-up<br>- 3 Mile Run<br>  - Moderate Effort<br>- Cool Down / Stretch | **AMRAP- 12 MINUTES**<br>- 5 Pull ups<br>- 10 Pushups<br>- 15 Squats | - OFF |
| **TUESDAY** | - OFF | **Complete 5 Rounds for Time**<br>- 15 DIAMOND PUSHUPS<br>- 20 METER BEAR CRAWL<br>- 15 MODIFIED V-SITS<br>- 10 DIPS<br>- 6 GLUTE HAM RAISES<br>- 10 PLANK REACHES | **WARM UP:**<br>- 300m kick, bottom arm out straight (no fins)<br>**MAIN SET:**<br>- 2 x 500m Freestyle (fins), 70-80% effort, 3 min rest<br>**COOL DOWN:** 200m Freestyle, easy<br>**TOTAL:** 1500m |
| **WEDNESDAY** | - Dynamic Warm-up<br>- Interval Workout 2<br>  - Reference Interval Generator for times<br>- Cool Down / Stretch | - OFF | **WARM UP:**<br>- 300m kick, bottom arm out straight (no fins)<br>- 200m Freestyle, easy<br>**MAIN SET:**<br>- 4 x 50m Freestyle (fins), 95% effort, 30 sec rest<br>- 2 x 500m Freestyle (No fins), 70-80% effort, 3 min rest<br>**COOL DOWN:** 100m Freestyle, easy<br>**TOTAL:** 1800m |
| **THURSDAY** | - OFF | **AMRAP-30 MINUTES**<br>- 6 CHIN UPS<br>- 5 PLYO SPLIT SQUAT<br>- 5 TOES TO BAR<br>- 6 ALTERNATING GRIP PULL UPS<br>- 15 AIR SQUATS<br>- 20 FLUTTER KICKS (4 count)<br>- 12 UNDERHAND BODYWEIGHT ROWS<br>- 8 REVERSE LUNGE (each side)<br>- 25 BICYCLES (4 count) | - OFF |
| **FRIDAY** | - Dynamic Warm-up<br>- Timed 1 ¼ Mile<br>  - Max Effort<br>- Cool Down / Stretch | **Complete 3 Rounds**<br>- 10 GLUTE BRIDES<br>- 25 PUSHUPS<br>- 25 LEG LIFTS<br>- 10 DONKEY KICKS (each leg)<br>- 6 DROP PUSHUPS<br>- 10 RUSSIAN TWISTS (4 count)<br>- 10 BODYWEIGHT DEEP SQUATS<br>- 10 DECLINE PUSHUPS<br>- 10 PLANK REACHES | - OFF |
| **SATURDAY** | - OFF | **Complete 3 Rounds**<br>- 20 AIR SQUATS<br>- 20 SECOND SQUAT HOLD<br>- 400 METER RUN | **WARM UP:**<br>- 200m kick, bottom arm out straight (no fins)<br>- 200m Freestyle, easy<br>**MAIN SET:**<br>- 4 x 50m Freestyle (fins), 95% effort, 30 sec rest<br>- 2 x 500m Freestyle (fins), 70-80% effort, 3 min rest<br>**COOL DOWN:** 200m Freestyle (No fins), easy<br>**TOTAL:** 1800m |
| **SUNDAY** | - OFF | OFF | - OFF |

# PHASE 1 WORKOUT
## WEEK 3 OF 11

| | CARDIO | PHYSICAL TRAINING | SWIM |
|---|---|---|---|
| **MONDAY** | - Dynamic Warm-up<br>- Timed Run<br>  - 30-40 min<br>  - Moderate Effort<br>- Cool Down / Stretch | **Complete 4 Rounds**<br>- 5 PULL UPS<br>- 10 PUSHUPS<br>- 20 SIT UPS<br>- 30 AIR SQUATS | OFF |
| **TUESDAY** | - OFF | **3 Rounds for time**<br>- 8 PLYO SPLIT SQUATS<br>- 15 BURPEES<br>- 60 SECOND PLANK<br>- 10 PULL UPS<br>- 25 PUSH UPS<br>- 60 SECOND LEFT SIDE PLANK<br>- 60 SECOND RIGHT SIDE PLANK<br>- 25 DECLINE PUSHUPS<br>- 10 DECLINE DIAMOND PUSHUPS<br>- 50 METER LUNGE WALK | **WARM UP:**<br>- 100m kick, bottom arm out straight (no fins)<br>- 100m Freestyle, easy<br>**MAIN SET:**<br>- 2 x 500m Freestyle (fins), 70-80% effort, 1 minute rest<br>**COOL DOWN:** 100m Freestyle, easy<br>**TOTAL:** 1300m |
| **WEDNESDAY** | - Dynamic Warm-up<br>- Interval Workout 3<br>  - Reference Interval Generator for times<br>- Cool Down / Stretch | - OFF | |
| **THURSDAY** | - OFF | **AMRAP 20 MINUTES**<br>- 5 CHEST TO BAR PULL UPS<br>- 10 LEG RAISES<br>- 10 MOUNTAIN CLIMBERS (4 count)<br>- 5 CHIN UPS<br>- 10 RUSSIAN TWISTS (4 count)<br>- 5 PLYO SPLIT SQUAT | **WARM UP: PM**<br>- 300m kick, bottom arm out straight (no fins)<br>- 300 m Freestyle, easy<br>**MAIN SET:**<br>- 4 x 50m Freestyle (No fins), 95% effort, 30 sec rest<br>- 2 x 500m Freestyle (No fins), 70-80% effort, 3 min rest<br>**COOL DOWN:** 200m Freestyle (fins), easy<br>**TOTAL:** 2000m |
| **FRIDAY** | - Dynamic Warm-up<br>- Timed 1 ½ Mile<br>  - Max Effort<br>- Cool Down / Stretch | **AMRAP 45 minutes**<br>- 15 AIR SQUATS<br>- 15 SHOULDER PUSHUPS<br>- 20 CAN CAN ABS<br>- 10 SLIDING LEG CURLS<br>- 20 SHOULDER CIRCLES (4 count)<br>- 10 MODIFIED V-SITS<br>- 10 TIPPING BIRD (each leg)<br>- 10 DIVE BOMBER PUSHUPS<br>- 10 RUSSIAN TWISTS (4 count)<br>- 15 CALF RAISES (each leg)<br>- 25 ARM FLUTTER KICKS (4 count)<br>- 8 SCORPIONS (each side) | OFF |
| **SATURDAY** | - OFF | **Complete 4 Rounds for Time**<br>- 400 METER RUN<br>- 20 BURPEES<br>- 15 PULL UPS | **WARM UP:**<br>- 100m kick, bottom arm out straight (no fins)<br>- 100m Freestyle, easy<br>**MAIN SET:**<br>- 2 x 500m Freestyle (fins), 70-80% effort, 30 sec rest<br>**COOL DOWN:** 100m Freestyle (fins), easy<br>**TOTAL:** 1300m |
| **SUNDAY** | - OFF | OFF | OFF |

# PHASE 1 WORKOUT
## WEEK 4 OF 11

|  | CARDIO | PHYSICAL TRAINING | SWIM |
|---|---|---|---|
| **MONDAY** | - Dynamic Warm-up<br>- 3 Mile Run<br>  - Moderate Effort<br>- Cool Down / Stretch | **Complete 3 Rounds**<br>- 20 METER BEAR CRAWL<br>- 25 SQUAT<br>- 20 METER CRAB WALK<br>- 10 REVERSE LUNGE (EACH SIDE)<br>- 10 METER INCHWORM<br>- 15 DIAMOND PUSHUPS | - OFF |
| **TUESDAY** | - OFF | **AMRAP 45 minutes**<br>- 15 PUSHUPS<br>- 6 CHIN UPS<br>- 12 MODIFIED VSITS<br>- 10 CLAPPING PUSHUPS<br>- 6 ALTERNATING GRIP PULL UPS<br>- 20 FLUTTER KICKS (4 count)<br>- 10 DECLINE PUSHUPS<br>- 10 UNDERHAND BODYWEIGHT ROWS<br>- 14 PLANK REACHES<br>- 10 WIDE PUSHUPS<br>- 8 ONE ARM SELF RESISTANT CURLS (each arm)<br>- 30 SECOND SIDE PLANKS (each side) | **WARM UP:**<br>- 100m kick, bottom arm out straight<br>- 100m Freestyle, easy<br>**MAIN SET:**<br>- 2 x 50m Freestyle (fins), 95% effort, 30 sec rest<br>- 2 x 400m Freestyle (fins), 70-80% effort, 3 min rest<br>**COOL DOWN:** 100m Freestyle, easy<br>**TOTAL:** 1300m |
| **WEDNESDAY** | - Dynamic Warm-up<br>- Interval Workout 4<br>  - Reference Interval Generator for times<br>- Cool Down / Stretch | - OFF | **PM**<br>**WARM UP:**<br>- 200m kick, bottom arm out straight<br>- 200m Freestyle, easy<br>**MAIN SET:**<br>- 6 x 50m Freestyle (fins), 95% effort, 30 sec rest<br>- 3 x 400m Freestyle (No fins), 70-80% effort, 3 min rest<br>**COOL DOWN:** 100m Freestyle, easy<br>**TOTAL:** 2000m |
| **THURSDAY** | - OFF | **EVERY MINUTE ON THE MINUTE (EMOM) FOR 20 MINUTES**<br>- 5 PULL UPS<br>- 5 PUSH UPS<br>- 10 SIT UPS | - OFF |
| **FRIDAY** | - Dynamic Warm-up<br>- Timed 1 ¾ Mile<br>  - Max Effort<br>- Cool Down / Stretch | **Complete 3 Rounds for Time**<br>- 25 SHOULDER CIRCLES (4 count; ea direction)<br>- 10 GLUTE HAM RAISE<br>- 20 POWER KNEES (each side)<br>- 20 DIPS<br>- 12 SINGLE LEG SLIDING LEG CURLS (each side)<br>- 40 SECOND SIDE PLANKS (each side)<br>- 15 SHOULDER PUSHUPS<br>- 20 DIAMOND PUSHUPS<br>- 10 MOUNTAIN CLIMBERS (4 count)<br>- 10 TIPPING BIRDS (each side)<br>- 12 DIVE BOMBERS<br>- 10 JUMPING JACKS (4 count) | - OFF |
| **SATURDAY** | - OFF | - OFF | **WARM UP:**<br>- 100m kick, bottom arm out straight (no fins)<br>- 100m Freestyle, easy<br>**MAIN SET:**<br>- 4 x 50m Freestyle (No fins), 95% effort, 30 sec rest<br>- 2 x 500m Freestyle (fins), 70-80% effort, 2 min rest<br>**COOL DOWN:** 200m Freestyle, easy<br>**TOTAL:** 1600m |
| **SUNDAY** | - OFF | - OFF | - OFF |

# PHASE 1 WORKOUT
## WEEK 5 OF 11

| | CARDIO | PHYSICAL TRAINING | SWIM |
|---|---|---|---|
| **MONDAY** | - Dynamic Warm-up<br>- 3 Mile Run<br>  - Moderate Effort<br>- Cool Down / Stretch | **MAX EFFORT 2 ROUNDS**<br>- PULL UPS in 1 minute<br>  2 minute rest<br>- SIT UPS in 2 minutes<br>  2 minute rest<br>- PUSHUPS in 2 minutes<br>  2 minute rest | - OFF |
| **TUESDAY** | - OFF | **Complete 3 Rounds for Time**<br>- 15 AIR SQUATS<br>- 30 SECOND FOREARM PLANK<br>- 10 BURPEES<br>- SIDE LUNGES (5ea LEG)<br>- 30 SECOND SIDE PLANK (each side)<br>- 10 SQUAT JUMPS<br>- 5 TOES TO BAR | **WARM UP:**<br>- 100m kick, bottom arm out straight (fins)<br>- 100m Freestyle, easy (fins)<br>**MAIN SET:**<br>- 4 x 50 m Freestyle (No fins), 95% effort, 30 sec rest<br>- 2 x 400m Freestyle (fins), 70-80% effort, 3 minute rest<br>**COOL DOWN:** 100m Freestyle, easy<br>**TOTAL:** 1300m |
| **WEDNESDAY** | - Dynamic Warm-up<br>- Interval Workout 4<br>  - Reference Interval Generator for times<br>- Cool Down / Stretch | - OFF | **PM**<br>**WARM UP:**<br>- 300m kick, bottom arm out straight<br>- 300m Freestyle, easy<br>**MAIN SET:**<br>- 3 x 400m Freestyle (No fins), 4 min rest<br>- 6 x 50m Freestyle (fins), 95% effort, 30 sec rest<br>**COOL DOWN:** 200m Freestyle, easy<br>**TOTAL:** 2300m |
| **THURSDAY** | - OFF | **AMRAP 30 MINUTES**<br>- 15 DIAMOND PUSH UPS<br>- 10 SIDE LUNGE (each side)<br>- 10 MOUNTAIN CLIMBERS<br>- 10 DIVE BOMBER PUSHUPS<br>- 8 SINGLE LEG SQUATS (each leg)<br>- 10 ONLIQUE V-UPS (each side)<br>- 10 SQUAT JUMPS<br>- 15 DIPS<br>- 25 BICYCLES (4 count) | - OFF |
| **FRIDAY** | - Dynamic Warm-up<br>- Timed 2 Mile<br>  - Max Effort<br>- Cool Down / Stretch | **Complete 3 Rounds for Time**<br>- 10 BURPEES<br>- 12 CHIN UPS<br>- 20 UNSUPPORTED SIT UPS<br>- 20 WIDE PUSHUPS<br>- 10 EXPLOSIVE PULL UPS WITH GRIP SWITCH<br>- 10 V-UPS<br>- 10 CLAPPING PUSHUPS<br>- 5 WIDE GRIP PULL UPS<br>- 10 OBLIQUE V-UPS<br>- 15 DECLINE PUSHUPS<br>- 15 UNDERHAND BODYWEIGHT ROWS<br>- 20 CAN CAN ABS | - OFF |
| **SATURDAY** | - OFF | **AMRAP 15 Minutes**<br>- 10 RFE SPLIT SQUAT (EACH)<br>- 10 PLYO INCLINE DIAMOND PUSHUPS<br>- 25 AIR SQUATS<br>- 10 PLYO PUSHUPS | **WARM UP:**<br>- 100m kick, bottom arm out straight<br>- 100m Freestyle, easy<br>**MAIN SET:**<br>- 4 x 50 m Freestyle, (fins) 95% effort, 30 sec rest<br>- 2 x 400m Freestyle (fins), 70-80% effort, 3 min rest<br>**COOL DOWN:** 100m Freestyle, easy<br>**TOTAL:** 1300m |
| **SUNDAY** | - OFF | - OFF | - OFF |

# PHASE 1 WORKOUT
## WEEK 6 OF 11

| | CARDIO | PHYSICAL TRAINING | SWIM |
|---|---|---|---|
| **MONDAY** | - OFF | **AMRAP 45 minutes**<br>- 15 PUSHUPS<br>- 6 CHIN UPS<br>- 12 MODIFIED VSITS<br>- 10 CLAPPING PUSHUPS<br>- 6 ALTERNATING GRIP PULL UPS<br>- 20 FLUTTER KICKS (4 count)<br>- 10 DECLINE PUSHUPS<br>- 15 UNDERHAND BODYWEIGHT ROWS<br>- 14 PLANK REACHES<br>- 10 WIDE PUSHUPS<br>- 8 UNEVEN PULL UPS<br>- 30 SECOND SIDE PLANKS (each side) | - OFF |
| **TUESDAY** | - Dynamic Warm-up<br>- Run for 3:00 min<br>- Sprints<br>  - 6 x 200m at <45 sec pace, rest 90 sec between runs<br>- Run for 3:00 min<br>- Cool Down/Stretch | - OFF | **WARM UP:**<br>- 100m kick, bottom arm out straight<br>- 100m Freestyle, easy<br>**MAIN SET:**<br>- 6 x 50m Freestyle (fins), 95% effort, 30 sec rest<br>- 1 x 400m Freestyle, 70-80% effort, 2 min rest<br>**COOL DOWN:** 100m Freestyle, easy<br>**TOTAL:** 1300m |
| **WEDNESDAY** | - OFF | **Complete 3 Rounds**<br>- 50 FLUTTER KICKS (4 count)<br>- 20 PUSH UPS<br>- 15 PULL UPS<br>- 30 BICYCLES (4 count)<br>- 10 DIPS<br>- 10 UNDERHAND BODYWEIGHT ROWS | **WARM UP:**<br>- 300m kick, bottom arm out straight<br>- 100m Freestyle, easy<br>**MAIN SET:**<br>- 6 x 50m Freestyle, 95% effort, 30 sec rest<br>- 3 x 400m Freestyle (fins), 70-80% effort, 3 minute rest<br>**COOL DOWN:** 100m Freestyle, easy<br>**TOTAL:** 2000m |
| **THURSDAY** | - Dynamic Warm-up<br>- 30 min run @ 60% effort<br>  - Increase to 80-90% for 30 sec every 2 min<br>- Cool Down / Stretch | - OFF | - OFF |
| **FRIDAY** | - OFF | **Complete 1 Round**<br>- ½ MILE JOG WARMUP<br>- ALTERNATE NEXT TWO EXERCISES UNTIL A TOTAL OF 800 METERS IS REACHED<br>- 100 METER SPRINT<br>- 100 METER LUNGE WALK<br>- 50 PULLUPS AS MANY SETS AS NECESSARY<br>- 800 METER RUN<br>- 50 VUPS<br>- 50 HANGING KNEES TO ELBOWS<br>- 800 METER COOL DOWN | - OFF |
| **SATURDAY** | - Dynamic Warm-up<br>- Sprints 12 x 100m at <20 sec, rest 25 sec between runs<br>- Run for 5:00 min<br>- Cool down/Stretch | - OFF | **WARM UP:**<br>- 200m kick, bottom arm out straight<br>- 100m Freestyle, easy<br>**MAIN SET:**<br>- 4 x 50m Freestyle (fins), 95% effort, 30 sec rest<br>- 2 x 400m Freestyle (fins), 70-80% effort, 2 min rest<br>**COOL DOWN:** 200m Freestyle, easy<br>**TOTAL:** 1500m |
| **SUNDAY** | - OFF | - OFF | - OFF |

# PHASE 1 WORKOUT
## WEEK 7 OF 11

| | CARDIO | PHYSICAL TRAINING | SWIM |
|---|---|---|---|
| **MONDAY** | o OFF | o 20 PUSH UPS<br>o 25 SIT UPS<br>o 10 CHIN UPS<br>o 25 FLUTTER KICKS (4 count)<br>o 15 DECLINE PUSHUPS<br>o 20 LEG RAISES<br>o 15 UNDERHAND BODYWEIGHT ROWS<br>o 20 SCISSORS<br>o 8 EXPLOSIVE PULL UPS WITH GRIP SWITCH<br>o 30 SECOND SIDE PLANK<br>o 25 BICYCLES (4 count) | o OFF |
| **TUESDAY** | o Dynamic Warm-up<br><br>o Timed 1-mile<br>• Max Effort<br>• Input results into Interval Workout in the "1 mile Re-Assessment Block"<br><br>o Cool Down / Stretch | o OFF | o OFF |
| **WEDNESDAY** | o OFF | **Complete 3 Rounds for Time**<br>o 15 BURPEES<br>o 12 PULL UPS<br>o 1 MINUTE PLANKS<br>o 15 CLAPPING PUSHUPS<br>o 15 BODYWEIGHT ROWS<br>o 10 WICKED WIPERS (4 count)<br>o 12 ROCKY PUSHUPS<br>o 10 WIDE GRIP PULL UPS<br>o 45 SECOND L-SIT<br>o 35 PUSHUPS<br>o 10 FRONT LEVERS (1 second holds)<br>o 20 LEG RAISES | **WARM UP:**<br>o 300m kick, bottom arm out straight (no fins)<br>o 100m Freestyle, easy<br>**MAIN SET:**<br>o 4 x 100m Freestyle (no fins), 95% effort, 1 min rest<br>o 2 x 600m Freestyle (fins), 70-80% effort, 4 min rest<br>**COOL DOWN:** 200m Freestyle, easy<br>**TOTAL:** 2200m |
| **THURSDAY** | o Dynamic Warm-up<br><br>o Interval Workout 5<br>• Reference Interval Generator for times<br><br>o Cool Down / Stretch | o OFF | **WARM UP:**<br>o 100m kick, bottom arm out straight (no fins)<br>o 100m Freestyle, easy (fins)<br>**MAIN SET:**<br>o 2 x 100m Freestyle (no fins), 95% effort, 1 min rest<br>o 1 x 600m Freestyle (fins), 70-80% effort, 4 min rest<br>**COOL DOWN:** 100m Freestyle, easy<br>**TOTAL:** 1100m |
| **FRIDAY** | o OFF | **Complete 3 Rounds for Time**<br>o 20 METER BEAR CRAWL<br>o 45 PUSHUPS<br>o 20 METER LUNGE WALK<br>o 60 SIT UPS<br>o 20 METER BROAD JUMPS<br>o 45 DIAMOND PUSHUPS<br>o 20 METERS CRAB CRAWL | OFF |
| **SATURDAY** | o Dynamic Warm-up<br>o 4 Mile Run<br>• Moderate Effort<br>o Cool Down / Stretch | OFF | **[Optional SWIM]**<br>**WARM UP:**<br>o 300m kick, bottom arm out straight (no fins)<br>o 300m Freestyle, easy<br>**MAIN SET:**<br>o 2 x 100m Freestyle (no fins), 95% effort, 1 min rest<br>o 2 x 600m Freestyle (fins), 70-80% effort, 4 min rest<br>**COOL DOWN:** 100m Freestyle (fins), easy<br>**TOTAL:** 2100m |
| **SUNDAY** | o OFF | OFF | OFF |

# PHASE 1 WORKOUT
## WEEK 8 OF 11

|  | **CARDIO** | **PHYSICAL TRAINING** | **SWIM** |
|---|---|---|---|
| **MONDAY** | o OFF | **5 Rounds for Time**<br>o 20 PULL UPS<br>o 30 PUSH UPS<br>o 40 SIT UPS<br>o 50 AIR SQUATS<br><br>REST 3 MINUTES BETWEEN ROUNDS ADD TIMES FROM EACH ROUND TO GET TOTAL TIME | **WARM UP:**<br>o 200m kick, bottom arm out straight (no fins)<br>o 100m Freestyle, easy<br>**MAIN SET:**<br>o 1 x 600m Freestyle, (fins) 70-80% effort, 3 min rest<br>o 2 x 100m Freestyle (no fins), 95% effort, 1 min rest<br>**COOL DOWN:** 200m Freestyle, easy<br>**TOTAL:** 1300m |
| **TUESDAY** | o Dynamic Warm-up<br>o Timed 2 Mile<br>  • Max Effort<br>o Cool Down / Stretch | o OFF | o OFF |
| **WEDNESDAY** | o OFF | **Complete 3 Rounds**<br>o 15 AIR SQUATS<br>o 30 SECOND FOREARM PLANK<br>o 10 BURPEES<br>o SIDE LUNGES (5ea LEG)<br>o 30 SECOND SIDE PLANK (each side)<br>o 10 SQUAT JUMPS<br>o 5 TOES TO BAR | o OFF |
| **THURSDAY** | o Dynamic Warm-up<br>o Interval Workout 6<br>  • Reference Interval Generator for times<br>o Cool Down / Stretch | o OFF | **WARM UP:**<br>o 300m kick, bottom arm out straight (no fins)<br>o 300m Freestyle, easy (fins)<br>**MAIN SET:**<br>o 4 x 100m Freestyle (no fins), 95% effort, 1 min rest<br>o 1 x 600m Freestyle (fins), 70-80% effort, 4 min rest<br>**COOL DOWN:** 200m Freestyle (fins), easy<br>**TOTAL:** 1800m |
| **FRIDAY** | o OFF | **AS MANY ROUNDS AS POSSIBLE (AMRAP) IN 20 MINUTES**<br>o 10 CHEST TO BAR PULL UPS<br>o 10 LEG RAISES<br>o 10 MOUNTAIN CLIMBERS (4 count)<br>o 10 CHIN UPS<br>o 10 RUSSIAN TWISTS (4 count)<br>o 10 PLYO SPLIT SQUAT | o OFF |
| **SATURDAY** | o Dynamic Warm-up<br>o 4 Mile Run<br>  • Moderate Effort<br>o Cool Down / Stretch | o OFF | **[Optional SWIM]**<br>**WARM UP:**<br>o 300m kick, bottom arm out straight (no fins)<br>o 300m Freestyle, easy<br>**MAIN SET:**<br>o 2 x 600m Freestyle (fins), 70-80% effort, 4 min rest<br>o 4 x 100m Freestyle (no fins), 95% effort, 70 sec rest<br>**COOL DOWN:** 200m Freestyle, easy<br>**TOTAL:** 2400m |
| **SUNDAY** | o OFF | o OFF | o OFF |

# PHASE 1 WORKOUT
## WEEK 9 OF 11

| | CARDIO | PHYSICAL TRAINING | SWIM |
|---|---|---|---|
| **MONDAY** | - OFF | **Complete 3 Rounds for Time**<br>- 15 ONE LEG GLUTE BRIDGE (EACH LEG)<br>- 10 CHIN UPS<br>- 15 V-UPS<br>- 25 CALF RAISES<br>- 15 UNDERHAND BODYWEIGHT ROWS<br>- 35 BICYCLES (4 count)<br>- 15 AIR SQUATS<br>- 20 PIGEON TOED CALF RAISES<br>- 20 PLANK REACHES<br>- 6 EXPLOSIVE PULL UPS WITH GRIP SWITCH<br>- 12 STEP UPS (each leg)<br>- 15 MOUNTAIN CLIMBERS (4 count) | - OFF |
| **TUESDAY** | - Dynamic Warm-up<br>- Timed 2 1/4 Mile<br>  - Max Effort<br>- Cool Down / Stretch | **Complete 3 Rounds for Time**<br>- 25 SHOULDER CIRCLES (4 count; ea direction)<br>- 10 GLUTE HAM RAISE<br>- 20 POWER KNEES (each side)<br>- 20 DIPS<br>- 12 SINGLE LEG SLIDING LEG CURLS (each side)<br>- 40 SECOND SIDE PLANKS (each side)<br>- 15 SHOULDER PUSHUPS<br>- 20 DIAMOND PUSHUPS<br>- 10 MOUNTAIN CLIMBERS (4 count)<br>- 10 TIPPING BIRDS (each side)<br>- 12 DIVE BOMBERS<br>- 10 JUMPING JACKS (4 count) | - OFF |
| **WEDNESDAY** | - OFF | - OFF | **WARM UP:**<br>- 300m kick, bottom arm out straight (no fins)<br>- 300m Freestyle, easy (fins)<br>**MAIN SET:**<br>- 4 x 100m Freestyle (no fins), 95% effort, 1 min rest<br>- 2 x 600m Freestyle (fins), 70-80% effort, 3 min rest<br>**COOL DOWN:** 200m Freestyle (fins), easy<br>**TOTAL:** 2400m |
| **THURSDAY** | - Dynamic Warm-up<br>- Interval Workout 7<br>  - Reference Interval Generator for times<br>- Cool Down / Stretch | **Complete 3 Rounds for Time**<br>- 35 PUSHUPS<br>- 8 PULL UPS<br>- 35 FLUTTER KICKS (4 count)<br>- 12 PLYO SPLIT SQUATS (4 count)<br>- 20 SWIMMERS<br>- 15 MOUNTAIN CLIMBERS (4 count)<br>- 15 BODYWEIGHT SISSY SQUATS<br>- 22 DECLINE PUSHUPS<br>- 10 RESISTANCE BAND CHOPS (each side)<br>- 35 BICYCLES (4 count)<br>- 10 CHAIR CLIMBS<br>- 20 POWER KNEES (each side) | **WARM UP:**<br>- 100m kick, bottom arm out straight (no fins)<br>- 100m Freestyle, easy (fins)<br>**MAIN SET:**<br>- 1 x 100m Freestyle (no fins), 95% effort, 30 sec rest<br>- 1 x 600m Freestyle (fins), 80% effort, 3 min rest<br>**COOL DOWN:** 100m Freestyle (fins), easy<br>**TOTAL:** 1000m |
| **FRIDAY** | - OFF | **AMRAP 45 minutes**<br>- 25 PUSHUPS<br>- 8 CHIN UPS<br>- 15 MODIFIED V-SITS<br>- 12 CLAPPING PUSHUPS<br>- 6 ALTERNATING GRIP PULL UPS<br>- 30 FLUTTER KICKS (4 count)<br>- 15 DECLINE PUSHUPS<br>- 15 UNDERHAND BODYWEIGHT ROWS<br>- 16 PLANK REACHES<br>- 15 WIDE PUSHUPS<br>- 8 UNEVEN PULL UPS (each arm)<br>- 30 SECOND SIDE PLANKS (each side) | - OFF |
| **SATURDAY** | - Dynamic Warm-up<br>- 4 Mile Run<br>  - Moderate Effort<br>- Cool Down / Stretch | - OFF | **WARM UP:**<br>- 300m kick, bottom arm out straight (no fins)<br>- 200m Freestyle, easy (fins)<br>**MAIN SET:**<br>- 4 x 100m Freestyle (no fins), 95% effort, 30 sec rest<br>- 2 x 600m Freestyle (fins), 70-80% effort, 3 min rest<br>**COOL DOWN:** 100m Freestyle (No fins), easy<br>**TOTAL:** 2200m |
| **SUNDAY** | - OFF | - OFF | - OFF |

# PHASE 1 WORKOUT
## WEEK 10 OF 11

| | CARDIO | PHYSICAL TRAINING | SWIM |
|---|---|---|---|
| **MONDAY** | - OFF | **Complete 3 Rounds for Time**<br>- 15 BURPEES<br>- 12 PULL UPS<br>- 1 MINUTE 30 SECOND PLANKS<br>- 15 CLAPPING PUSHUPS<br>- 20 BODYWEIGHT ROWS<br>- 8 WICKED WIPERS (4 count)<br>- 12 ROCKY PUSHUPS<br>- 15 WIDE GRIP PULL UPS<br>- 45 SECOND L-SIT<br>- 35 PUSHUPS<br>- 10 FRONT LEVERS (1 second holds)<br>- 30 LEG RAISES | - OFF |
| **TUESDAY** | - Dynamic Warm-up<br>- Timed 2 1/2 Mile<br>  • Max Effort<br>- Cool Down / Stretch | **Complete 3 Rounds for Time**<br>- 15 CHIN UPS<br>- 20 BODYWEIGHT TRICEPS EXTENSIONS<br>- 30 BICYCLES (4 count)<br>- 15 UNDERHAND BODYWEIGHT ROWS<br>- 10 DIPS<br>- 30 BICYCLES (4 count)<br>- 10 ALTERNATING PULL UPS WITH GRIP SWITCH<br>- 20 MODIFIED V-SITS<br>- 5 UNEVEN PULL UPS<br>- 25 DIAMOND PUSHUPS<br>- 15 MOUNTAIN CLIMBERS (4 count) | **WARM UP:**<br>- 400m kick, bottom arm out straight<br>- 400m Freestyle, easy<br>**MAIN SET:**<br>- 4 x 100m Freestyle (fins), 95% effort, 1 min rest<br>- 1 x 1000m Freestyle (fins), 70-80% effort, 5 min rest<br>**COOL DOWN:** 200m Freestyle (No fins), easy<br>**TOTAL:** 2300m |
| **WEDNESDAY** | - OFF | - OFF | **WARM UP:**<br>- 100m kick, bottom arm out straight<br>- 100m Freestyle, easy<br>**MAIN SET:**<br>- 6 x 100m Freestyle (fins), 95% effort, 30 sec rest<br>- 1 x 800m Freestyle (fins), 70-80% effort, 4 min rest<br>**COOL DOWN:** 100m Freestyle, easy<br>**TOTAL:** 1700m |
| **THURSDAY** | - Dynamic Warm-up<br>- Interval Workout 8<br>  • Reference Interval Generator for times<br>- Cool Down / Stretch | **Complete 3 Rounds for Time**<br>- 20 AIR SQUATS<br>- 20 SHOULDER PUSHUPS<br>- 30 FLUTTER KICKS (4 count)<br>- 10 TWISTING LUNGES (each leg)<br>- 10 HAND STAND PUSHUPS<br>- 30 BICYCLES (4 count)<br>- 10 ONE-LEG SQUATS (each leg)<br>- 15 DIVE BOMBER PUSHUPS<br>- 20 POWER KNEES (each side)<br>- 20 CALF RAISES (each leg)<br>- 20 METER HANDSTAND WALK<br>- 40 SECOND LSIT | OFF |
| **FRIDAY** | - OFF | **Complete 3 Rounds as Quickly as Possible**<br>- 15 BURPEES<br>- 12 CHIN UPS<br>- 25 UNSUPPORTED SIT UPS<br>- 30 WIDE PUSHUPS<br>- 10 EXPLOSIVE PULL UPS WITH GRIP SWITCH<br>- 15 V-UPS<br>- 15 CLAPPING PUSHUPS<br>- 10 ALTERNATING GRIP PULL UPS<br>- 10 OBLIQUE V-UPS (each side)<br>- 25 DECLINE PUSHUPS<br>- 15 UNDERHAND BODYWEIGHT ROWS<br>- 20 CAN CAN ABS | OFF |
| **SATURDAY** | - Dynamic Warm-up<br>- 4 Mile Run<br>  • Moderate Effort<br>- Cool Down / Stretch | OFF | **WARM UP:**<br>- 400m kick, bottom arm out straight (No fins)<br>- 200m Freestyle, easy (fins)<br>**MAIN SET:**<br>- 6 x 100m Freestyle (fins), 95% effort, 30 sec rest<br>- 1 x 1000m Freestyle (No fins), 70-80% effort, 2 min rest<br>**COOL DOWN:** 200m Freestyle (fins), easy<br>**TOTAL:** 2400m |
| **SUNDAY** | - OFF | OFF | OFF |

# PHASE 1 WORKOUT
## WEEK 11 OF 11

|  | CARDIO | PHYSICAL TRAINING | SWIM |
|---|---|---|---|
| **MONDAY** | PAST<br>*Record 1.5 mi time for Interval Generator for re-calculation | PAST<br>* | PAST<br>* |
| **TUESDAY** | o OFF | **5 Rounds for Time**<br>o 20 AIR SQUATS<br>o 20 PUSH UPS<br>o ALTERNATING LUNGES (10ea LEG)<br>o 10 SUPERMANS<br>o 10 V-UPS | **WARM UP:**<br>o 100m kick, bottom arm out straight<br>o 100m Freestyle, easy<br>**MAIN SET:**<br>o 2 x 100m Freestyle (fins), 95% effort, 30 sec rest<br>o 1 x 1000m Freestyle (fins), 70-80% effort, 3 min rest<br>**COOL DOWN:** 200m Freestyle, easy<br>**TOTAL:** 1600m |
| **WEDNESDAY** | o Dynamic Warm-up<br>o Interval Workout 1<br>• Reference Interval Generator for times<br>o Cool Down / Stretch | o OFF | o OFF |
| **THURSDAY** | o OFF | **AMRAP 20 MINUTES**<br>o 10 CHEST TO BAR PULL UPS<br>o 10 LEG RAISES<br>o 10 MOUNTAIN CLIMBERS (4 count)<br>o 10 CHIN UPS<br>o 10 RUSSIAN TWISTS (4 count)<br>o 10 PLYO SPLIT SQUAT | **WARM UP:**<br>o 200m kick, bottom arm out straight<br>o 200m Freestyle, easy<br>**MAIN SET:**<br>o 3 x 100m Freestyle (fins), 95% effort, 30 sec rest<br>o 1 x 800m Freestyle (fins), 70-80% effort, 3 min rest<br>**COOL DOWN:** 200m Freestyle, easy<br>**TOTAL:** 1600m |
| **FRIDAY** | o Dynamic Warm-up<br>o 4 ½ Mile Run<br>• Moderate Effort<br>o Cool Down / Stretch | **EVERY MINUTE ON THE MINUTE (EMOM) FOR 20 MINUTES**<br>o 5 PULL UPS<br>o 5 PUSH UPS<br>o 10 SIT UPS | o OFF |
| **SATURDAY** | o OFF | o OFF | **WARM UP:**<br>o 200m kick, bottom arm out straight<br>o 200m Freestyle, easy (fins)<br>**MAIN SET:**<br>o 6 x 100m Freestyle (fins), 95% effort, 30 sec rest<br>o 1 x 1000m Freestyle (fins), 70-80% effort, 3 min rest<br>**COOL DOWN:** 200m Freestyle, easy<br>**TOTAL:** 2200m |
| **SUNDAY** | o OFF | OFF | OFF |

| Insert most recent 1.5 mile assessment time in cell D2 below to obtain individual work interval times | | | | | | | | |
|---|---|---|---|---|---|---|---|---|
| Date | Name | 2400m | | **9:45** | 1600m | **6:30** | 6:02 | (=9:00 x 0.62) |
| | | | | | | | | |
| | **Track** | | | Work | Work:Rest | Rep Rest | Set Rest | Split | Split |
| **Workout Order** | **Workout** | Factor | | **Interval** | Ratio | Interval | Interval | | |
| | W-out volume | | | (mins) | | (mins) | (mins) | | |
| | | | | | | | | 200m | |
| 1 | **2 x 4 x 400m** | 0.975 | | **1:35** | 1:0.5 | 0:47 | 3:00 | 0:47 | |
| | 3200m | | | | | | | | |
| | | | | | | | | 400m | 800m |
| 2 | **1 x 3 x 1200m** | 1.05 | | **5:07** | 1:0.5 | 2:33 | na | 1:42 | 3:24 |
| | 3600m | | | | | | | | |
| | | | | | | | | 200m | 400m |
| 3 | **1 x 3 x 600m** | 0.97 | | **2:21** | 1:1 | 2:21 | 3:00 | 0:47 | 1:34 |
| | **1 x 3 x 200m** | 0.90 | | **0:43** | 1:1 | 0:43 | 3:00 | | |
| | **2 x 3 x 200m** | 0.85 | | **0:41** | 1:1.5 | 1:02 | 3:00 | | |
| | 3600m | | | | | | | | |
| | | | | | | | | 200m | 400m |
| 4 | **1 x 3 x 800m** | 0.97 | | **3:09** | 1:1 | 3:09 | 4:00 | 0:47 | 1:34 |
| | **1 x 4 x 400m** | 0.91 | | **1:28** | 1:1 | 1:28 | | 0:44 | |
| | 4000m | | | | | | | | |
| | | | | | | | | | |
| Perform a 1.0 mile reassessment between weeks 4 and 5 and enter new time below | | | | | | | | |
| Date | Name | | | | 1600m | **6:15** | (reassessment 1.0 time here) | | |
| | | | | | (1.0 mi) | | | | . |
| | | | | Work | Work:Rest | Rep Rest | Set Rest | Split | Split |
| **Workout Order** | **Workout** | Factor | | **Interval** | Ratio | Interval | Interval | | |
| | W-out | | | (mins) | | (mins) | (mins) | | |

| # | Workout | | | | | | 200m | 400m | | | |
|---|---|---|---|---|---|---|---|---|---|---|---|
| | volume | | | | | | | | | | |
| 5 | **1200m Aus Pursuit** | | **5:48** | | | | 0:58 | 1:56 | | | |
| | **1 x 3 x 600m** | 0.98 | **2:17** | 1:1 | 2:17 | 4:00 | 0:45 | 1:31 | | | |
| | **1 x 4 x 300m** | 0.91 | **1:03** | 1:1 | 1:03 | | 0:42 | | | | |
| | 4200m | | | | | | | | | | |
| 6 | **Newtons** | (same work time, decreasing rest time) | | | | | Rep restart times | | | | |
| | **4 x 5 x 200m** | 0.95 | **0:44** | decreasing | 45/35/25/15 | 2:00 | Set 1 | Set 2 | Set 3 | Set 4 | |
| | 4000m | | | | (secs) | | 1:30 | 1:20 | 1:10 | 1:00 | |
| | | | | | | | 200m | | | | |
| 7 | **Knockouts** | (run at one second + 400m time at 1600m race pace) | | | | | | | | | |
| | **1 x 10 x 400m** | 0:01 | **1:34** | ≈1:1 | 90 secs | | 0:47 | | | | |
| | 4000m | | 1:33 | | | | | | | | |
| | | | | | | 200m | | | | | |
| 8 | **2 x 4 x 400m** | | **1:33** | 1:0.5 | 0:46 | 3:00 | 0:46 | | | | |
| | 3200m | | | | | | | | | | |
| | Compare Workout 8 to Workout 1 - note your improvement | | | | | | | | | | |

Page 53

# PHASE 2 WORKOUT
## WEEK 1 OF 15

| | CARDIO | PHYSICAL TRAINING | SWIM |
|---|---|---|---|
| **MONDAY** | - Dynamic Warm-up<br>- Timed 2-3/4 Mile<br>  • Max Effort<br>- Cool Down / Stretch | **Complete 3 Rounds for Time**<br>- 10 HANDSTAND PUSHUPS<br>- 20 AIR SQUATS<br>- 50 FLUTTER KICKS (4 count)<br>- 25 SHOULDER PUSHUPS<br>- 15 SLIDING CURLS (each leg)<br>- 30 BICYCLES<br>- 40 ARM FLUTTER KICKS (4 count)<br>- 15 SISSY SQUATS<br>- 30 ROCKY SIT UPS<br>- 8 WALL WALKS<br>- 25 CALF RAISES (each side)<br>- 30 SECOND L-SIT | - OFF |
| **TUESDAY** | - OFF | **Complete 3 Rounds for Time**<br>- 15 UNDERHAND BODYWEIGHT ROWS<br>- 30 DIAMOND PUSH UPS<br>- 15 HANGING LEG RAISES<br>- 10 UNEVEN CHIN UPS (EACH ARM)<br>- 30 DIPS<br>- 50 BICYCLES (4 count)<br>- 15 CHIN UPS<br>- 20 BODYWEIGHT TRICEPS EXTENSIONS<br>- 30 ROCKY SIT UPS<br>- 12 ONE ARM UNDERHAND BODYWEIGHT ROWS<br>- 25 CLOSE GRIP PUSHUPS<br>- 15 POWER KNEES (each side) | **WARM UP:**<br>- 200m kick, bottom arm out straight<br>- 200m Freestyle, easy<br>**MAIN SET:**<br>- 6 x 100m Freestyle (No fins), 95% effort, 20 sec rest<br>- 1 x 1000m Freestyle (fins), 70-80% effort, 30 sec rest<br>**COOL DOWN:** 100m Freestyle, easy<br>**TOTAL: 2100m** |
| **WEDNESDAY** | - Dynamic Warm-up<br>- Interval Workout 2<br>  • Reference Interval Generator for times<br>- Cool Down / Stretch | - OFF | **WARM UP:**<br>- 200m kick, bottom arm out straight<br>- 100m Freestyle, easy<br>**MAIN SET:**<br>- 4 x 100m Freestyle (fins), 95% effort, 1 min rest<br>- 1 x 800m Freestyle (fins), 70-80% effort, 3 min rest<br>**COOL DOWN:** 100m Freestyle (fins), easy<br>**TOTAL: 1800m** |
| **THURSDAY** | - OFF | **Complete 3 Rounds for Time**<br>- 15 PULL UPS<br>- 35 PUSHUPS<br>- 10 V-UPS<br>- 15 BODYWEIGHT ROWS<br>- 12 ROCKY PUSHUPS<br>- 20 BICYCLES (4 count)<br>- 10 FRONT LEVERS<br>- 15 DROP PUSH UPS<br>- 20 PLANK REACHES<br>- 10 WIDE PULL UPS<br>- 10 CLAPPING PUSHUPS<br>- 10 FLOOR WIPERS (each side) | - OFF |
| **FRIDAY** | - Dynamic Warm-up<br>- 5 Mile Run<br>  • Moderate Effort<br>- Cool Down / Stretch | **Complete 3 Rounds for Time**<br>- 20 AIR SQUATS<br>- 15 CHIN UPS<br>- 15 HANGING LEG RAISES<br>- 25 CALF RAISES (each leg)<br>- 10 ONE ARM CHIN UPS (EACH ARM; ASSISTED)<br>- 50 BICYCLES (4 count)<br>- 10 ONE LEG SQUATS (each leg)<br>- 15 UNDERHAND BODYWEIGHT ROWS<br>- 20 VUPS<br>- 15 HAMSTRING CURLS (each leg)<br>- 25 UNDERHAND PUSHUPS<br>- 25 LEG RAISES | **WARM UP:**<br>- 200m kick, bottom arm out straight<br>- 100m Freestyle, easy<br>**MAIN SET:**<br>- 6 x 100m Freestyle (fins), 95% effort, 1 min rest<br>- 1 x 1000m Freestyle (No fins), 70-80% effort, 3 min rest<br>**COOL DOWN:** 200m Freestyle, easy<br>**TOTAL: 2600m** |
| **SATURDAY** | - OFF | **Complete 3 Rounds for Time**<br>- 50 PUSHUPS<br>- 25 DIAMOND PUSHUPS<br>- 50 FLUTTER KICKS (4 count)<br>- 35 DECLINE PUSHUPS<br>- 15 PLYO PUSHUPS<br>- 40 ROCKY SIT UPS<br>- 20 DIVE BOMBERS<br>- 10 CORN COB PUSHUPS<br>- 15 POWER KNEES (each side)<br>- 15 BURPEES<br>- 25 WIDE PUSHUPS<br>- 30 RUSSIAN TWISTS (4 count) | - OFF |
| **SUNDAY** | - OFF | - OFF | - OFF |

# PHASE 2 WORKOUT
## WEEK 2 OF 15

|  | CARDIO | PHYSICAL TRAINING | SWIM |
|---|---|---|---|
| **MONDAY** | - Dynamic Warm-up<br>- Timed 3 Mile<br>  - Max Effort<br>- Cool Down / Stretch | **AMRAP 45 minutes**<br>- 35 PUSHUPS<br>- 10 CHIN UPS<br>- 20 MODIFIED V-SITS<br>- 15 CLAPPING PUSHUPS<br>- 8 ALTERNATING GRIP PULL UPS<br>- 30 FLUTTER KICKS (4 count)<br>- 20 DECLINE PUSHUPS<br>- 15 UNDERHAND BODYWEIGHT ROWS<br>- 20 PLANK REACHES<br>- 20 WIDE PUSHUPS<br>- 8 UNEVEN PULL UPS (each arm)<br>- 30 SECOND SIDE PLANKS (each side) | - OFF |
| **TUESDAY** | - OFF | **Complete 3 Rounds for Time**<br>- 25 SHOULDER CIRCLES (4 count; ea direction)<br>- 10 GLUTE HAM RAISE<br>- 20 POWER KNEES (each side)<br>- 30 DIPS<br>- 12 SINGLE LEG SLIDING LEG CURLS (each side)<br>- 40 SECOND SIDE PLANKS (each side)<br>- 15 SHOULDER PUSHUPS<br>- 25 DIAMOND PUSHUPS<br>- 10 MOUNTAIN CLIMBERS (4 count)<br>- 10 TIPPING BIRDS (each side)<br>- 12 DIVE BOMBERS<br>- 10 JUMPING JACKS (4 count) | **WARM UP:**<br>- 200m Freestyle<br>- 200m Lead arm- Trail arm, easy (fins)<br>**MAIN SET:**<br>- 3 x 100m Lead arm- Trail arm (fins), 95% effort, 30 sec rest<br>- 1 x 1000m Lead arm- Trail arm (fins), 70-80% effort, 2 min rest<br>**COOL DOWN:** 100m Lead arm- Trail arm, easy<br>**TOTAL:** 1800m |
| **WEDNESDAY** | - Dynamic Warm-up<br>- Interval Workout 3<br>  - Reference Interval Generator for times<br>- Cool Down / Stretch | - OFF | **WARM UP:**<br>- 400m Freestyle<br>- 400m Lead arm- Trail arm, easy<br>**MAIN SET:**<br>- 3 x 100m Lead arm- Trail arm (fins), 95% effort, 1 min rest<br>- 1 x 1000m Lead arm- Trail arm (fins), 70-80% effort, 3 min rest<br>- 3 x 100m Lead arm- Trail arm, 70% effort, 30 sec rest<br>**COOL DOWN:** 200m Lead arm- Trail arm, easy<br>**TOTAL:** 2600m |
| **THURSDAY** | - OFF | **Complete 3 Rounds for time**<br>- 15 PLYO SPLIT SQUATS<br>- 50 DIAMOND PUSHUPS<br>- 1 MINUTE 30 SECOND PLANK<br>- 15 BODYWEIGHT SISSY SQUATS<br>- 40 DIPS<br>- 5 DRAGON FLAGS<br>- 15 ONE-LEG SQUATS (each leg)<br>- 25 SPHINX PUSHUPS<br>- 40 ROCKY SIT UPS<br>- 30 CALF RAISES<br>- 20 BODYWEIGHT TRICEPS EXTENSIONS<br>- 40 SECOND L-SIT | - OFF |
| **FRIDAY** | - Dynamic Warm-up<br>- 5 Mile Run<br>  - Moderate Effort<br>- Cool Down / Stretch | **EVERY MINUTE ON THE MINUTE (EMOM) FOR 20 MINUTES**<br>- 5 PULL UPS<br>- 5 PUSH UPS<br>- 10 SIT UPS | **WARM UP:**<br>- 200m Freestyle<br>- 200m Lead arm- Trail arm, easy (fins)<br>**MAIN SET:**<br>- 4 x 100m Lead arm- Trail arm (fins), 95% effort, 1 min rest<br>- 1 x 800m Lead arm- Trail arm (fins), 70-80% effort, 30 sec rest<br>**COOL DOWN:** 100m Lead arm- Trail arm, easy<br>**TOTAL:** 1700m |
| **SATURDAY** | - OFF | **AS MANY ROUNDS AS POSSIBLE (AMRAP) IN 20 MINUTES**<br>- 10 CHEST TO BAR PULL UPS<br>- 10 LEG RAISES<br>- 10 MOUNTAIN CLIMBERS (4 count)<br>- 10 CHIN UPS<br>- 10 RUSSIAN TWISTS (4 count)<br>- 10 PLYO SPLIT SQUAT | - OFF |
| **SUNDAY** | - OFF | - OFF | - OFF |

# PHASE 2 WORKOUT
## WEEK 3 OF 15

| | CARDIO | PHYSICAL TRAINING | SWIM |
|---|---|---|---|
| **MONDAY** | - Dynamic Warm-up<br>- Timed 3 Mile<br>  • Max Effort<br>- Cool Down / Stretch | **5 Rounds for Time**<br>- 20 PULL UPS<br>- 30 PUSH UPS<br>- 40 SIT UPS<br>- 50 AIR SQUATS<br><br>REST 3 MINUTES BETWEEN ROUNDS ADD TIMES FROM EACH ROUND TO GET TOTAL TIME | - OFF |
| **TUESDAY** | - OFF | **3 Rounds for Time**<br>- 20 METER BEAR CRAWL<br>- 25 SQUAT<br>- 20 METER CRAB CRAWL<br>- 10 REVERSE LUNGE (each side)<br>- 10 METER INCHWORM<br>- 15 DIAMOND PUSH UP | **WARM UP:**<br>- 200m Freestyle<br>**MAIN SET:**<br>- 3 x 100m Lead arm- Trail arm (fins), 95% effort, 30 sec rest<br>- 1 x 1000m Lead arm- Trail arm, 70-80% effort, 2 min rest<br>**COOL DOWN:** 100m Lead arm- Trail arm (fins), easy<br>**TOTAL:** 1600m |
| **WEDNESDAY** | - Dynamic Warm-up<br>- Interval Workout 4<br>  • Reference Interval Generator for times<br>- Cool Down / Stretch | - OFF | **WARM UP:**<br>- 300m Freestyle<br>**MAIN SET:**<br>- 4 x 100m Lead arm- Trail arm (fins), 95% effort, 1 min rest<br>- 1 x 1000m Lead arm- Trail arm (fins), 70-80% effort, 30 sec rest<br>**COOL DOWN:** 100m Lead arm- Trail arm (No fins), easy<br>**TOTAL:** 1800m |
| **THURSDAY** | - OFF | **Complete 3 Rounds for Time**<br>- 40 PUSHUPS<br>- 10 PULL UPS<br>- 35 FLUTTER KICKS (4 count)<br>- 12 PLYO SPLIT SQUATS (4 count)<br>- 20 SWIMMERS<br>- 15 MOUNTAIN CLIMBERS (4 count)<br>- 15 BODYWEIGHT SISSY SQUATS<br>- 25 DECLINE PUSHUPS<br>- 35 BICYCLES (4 count)<br>- 20 PLYO PUSHUPS<br>- 15 BODYWEIGHT ROWS<br>- 20 POWER KNEES (each side) | - OFF |
| **FRIDAY** | - Dynamic Warm-up<br>- 4 Mile Run<br>  • Moderate Effort<br>- Cool Down / Stretch | **Complete 3 Rounds for Time**<br>- 15 ONE LEG GLUTE BRIDGE (each leg)<br>- 10 CHIN UPS<br>- 15 V-UPS<br>- 25 CALF RAISES<br>- 15 UNDERHAND BODYWEIGHT ROWS<br>- 40 BICYCLES (4 count)<br>- 15 AIR SQUATS<br>- 20 PIGEON TOED CALF RAISES<br>- 20 PLANK REACHES<br>- 8 EXPLOSIVE PULL UPS WITH GRIP SWITCH<br>- 12 STEP UPS (each leg)<br>- 15 MOUNTAIN CLIMBERS (4 count) | **WARM UP:**<br>- 400m Freestyle<br>- 400m Lead arm- Trail arm, easy<br>**MAIN SET:**<br>- 4 x 100m Lead arm- Trail arm (fins), 95% effort, 1 min rest<br>- 1 x 1200m Lead arm- Trail arm (fins), 70-80% effort, 3 min rest<br>**COOL DOWN:** 200m Lead arm- Trail arm, easy<br>**TOTAL:** 2600m |
| **SATURDAY** | - OFF | **AMRAP 30 Minutes**<br>- 20 BODYWEIGHT TRICEPS EXTENSIONS<br>- 15 HANGING LEGRAISES<br>- 20 BODYWEIGHT ROWS<br>- 30 DIPS<br>- 50 BICYCLES (4 count)<br>- 15 FRONT LEVERS<br>- 20 VUPS<br>- 30 DIAMOND PUSHUPS<br>- 25 LEG RAISES | **WARM UP:**<br>- 1 x 400m Freestyle<br>- 1 x 400m Lead arm- Trail arm, easy (fins)<br>**MAIN SET:**<br>- 2 x 100m Lead arm- Trail arm, 95% effort, 20 sec rest<br>- 1 x 600m Lead arm- Trail arm, 70-80% effort, 30 sec rest<br>**COOL DOWN:** 100m Lead arm- Trail arm, easy<br>**TOTAL:** 1100m |
| **SUNDAY** | - OFF | - OFF | - OFF |

# PHASE 2 WORKOUT
## WEEK 4 OF 15

| | CARDIO | PHYSICAL TRAINING | SWIM |
|---|---|---|---|
| **MONDAY** | o OFF | **Complete 1 Round**<br>o ½ MILE JOG WARMUP<br>o ALTERNATE NEXT TWO EXERCISES UNTIL A TOTAL OF 800 METERS IS REACHED<br>o 100 METER SPRINT<br>o 100 METER LUNGE WALK<br><br>o 100 PULLUPS AS MANY SETS AS NECESSARY<br>o 800 METER RUN<br>o 75 VUPS<br>o 75 HANGING KNEES TO ELBOWS<br>o 800 METER COOL DOWN | o OFF |
| **TUESDAY** | o Dynamic Warm-up<br>o Timed Run<br>• 30-40 min<br>• Moderate Effort<br>o Cool Down / Stretch | **Complete 3 Rounds**<br>o 40 PUSHUPS<br>o 10 PULL UPS<br>o 35 FLUTTER KICKS (4 count)<br>o 12 PLYO SPLIT SQUATS (4 count)<br>o 20 SWIMMERS<br>o 15 MOUNTAIN CLIMBERS (4 count)<br>o 15 BODYWEIGHT SISSY SQUATS<br>o 22 DECLINE PUSHUPS<br>o 10 RESISTANCE BAND CHOPS (each side)<br>o 35 BICYCLES (4 count)<br>o 15 PLYO PUSHUPS<br>o 20 POWER KNEES (each side) | o OFF |
| **WEDNESDAY** | o OFF | o OFF | **WARM UP:**<br>o 800m Freestyle<br>**MAIN SET:**<br>o 3 x 100m Lead arm- Trail arm (fins), 95% effort, 1 min rest<br>o 1 x 1000m Lead arm- Trail arm (fins), 70 effort, 3 min rest<br>o 3x100m Lead arm- Trail arm (fins), 75% effort, 20 sec rest<br>**COOL DOWN:** 200m Lead arm- Trail arm, easy<br>**TOTAL: 2600m** |
| **THURSDAY** | o Dynamic Warm-up<br><br>o Sprints 12 x 100m at ~16 sec, rest 30 sec between runs<br><br>o Easy Run for 5:00 min<br><br>o Cool down/Stretch | **Complete 3 Rounds for Time**<br>o 10 Pull ups<br>o 25 Shoulder Circles (4 count)<br>o 30 Bicycles (4 count)<br>o 20 Swimmers<br>o 12 Dive Bombers<br>o 20 Rocky Sit ups<br>o 15 Bodyweight Rows<br>o 15 SHOULDER Pushups<br>o 15 Power Knees (each side)<br>o 15 Wide Pushups<br>o 8 Wide Pull ups<br>o 1 Minute Plank | o OFF |
| **FRIDAY** | o OFF | **5 Rounds for Time**<br>o 20 AIR SQUATS<br>o 20 PUSH UPS<br>o ALTERNATING LUNGES (10ea LEG)<br>o 10 SUPERMANS<br>o 10 V-UPS | **WARM UP:**<br>o 400m Freestyle<br>o 400m Lead arm- Trail arm, easy<br>**MAIN SET:**<br>o 6 x 100m Lead arm- Trail arm (fins), 95% effort, 90 sec rest<br>o 1 x 1000m Lead arm- Trail arm (fins), 70 effort, 2 min rest<br>**COOL DOWN:** 200m Lead arm- Trail arm (fins), easy<br>**TOTAL: 2600m** |
| **SATURDAY** | o Dynamic Warm-up<br>o 5 Mile Run<br>• Moderate Effort<br>o Cool Down / Stretch | **3 Rounds for time**<br>o 5 PLYO PUSH UP<br>o 5 PLYO SPLIT SQUAT (each leg)<br>o 5 L-SIT PULL UP<br>o 30 SEC PLANK<br>o 30 SECOND RIGHT SIDE PLANK<br>o 30 SECOND LEFT SIDE PLANK<br>o 10 JUMP SQUAT | **WARM UP:**<br>o 100m Freestyle<br>o 100m Lead arm- Trail arm, easy<br>**MAIN SET:**<br>o 3 x 100m Lead arm- Trail arm (fins), 95% effort, 1 min rest<br>o 1 x 800m Lead arm- Trail arm (fins), 70 effort, 3 min rest<br>**COOL DOWN:** 200m Lead arm- Trail arm, easy<br>**TOTAL: 1600m** |
| **SUNDAY** | o OFF | o OFF | o OFF |

# PHASE 2 WORKOUT
## WEEK 5 OF 15

| | CARDIO | PHYSICAL TRAINING | SWIM |
|---|---|---|---|
| **MONDAY** | - OFF | **Complete 3 Rounds for Time**<br>- 10 CHIN UPS<br>- 35 PUSHUPS<br>- 35 FLUTTER KICKS (4 count)<br>- 12 BODYWEIGHT BICEP CURLS<br>- 15 CLAPPING PUSHUPS<br>- 15 MODIFIED V-SITS<br>- 30 SECOND CHIN UP HOLDS<br>- 15 DIVE BOMBERS<br>- 35 BICYCLES (4 count)<br>- 15 UNDERHAND BODYWEIGHT ROWS<br>- 25 DECLINE PUSHUPS<br>- 15 POWER KNEES (each side) | - OFF |
| **TUESDAY** | - Dynamic Warm-up<br>- 4 Mile Run<br>  - Moderate Effort<br>- Cool Down / Stretch | - OFF | **WARM UP:**<br>- Freestyle<br>- 200m Lead arm- Trail arm, easy (fins)<br>**MAIN SET:**<br>- 3 x 200m Lead arm- Trail arm, 85% effort, 2 min rest<br>- 2 x 500m Lead arm- Trail arm (fins), 70 effort, 3 min rest<br>**COOL DOWN:** 100m Lead arm- Trail arm (fins), easy<br>**TOTAL: 2000m** |
| **WEDNESDAY** | - OFF | **Complete 3 Rounds for Time**<br>- 30 DIAMOND PUSHUPS<br>- 30 BODY SQUATS<br>- 15 RUSSIAN TWISTS (4 count)<br>- 15 DIPS<br>- 10 TWISTING LUNGES (each leg)<br>- 20 LEG RAISES<br>- 15 SPHINX PUSHUPS<br>- 25 METER CRABWALKS<br>- 30 SECOND L-SITS<br>- 15 BODYWEIGHT TRICEPS EXTENSIONS<br>- 25 CALF RAISES (each leg)<br>- 35 BICYCLES (4 count) | **WARM UP:**<br>- Freestyle<br>- 200m Lead arm- Trail arm, easy<br>**MAIN SET:**<br>- 2 x 500m Lead arm- Trail arm (fins), 85% effort, 30 sec rest<br>**COOL DOWN:** 100m Lead arm- Trail arm, easy<br>**TOTAL: 1600m** |
| **THURSDAY** | - Dynamic Warm-up<br>- Run 1 mile at 6:45 min pace<br>- Rest for 4 min<br>- Run 2 miles at 7:30 min pace, rest 5 min<br>- Run 1 mile at 7:00 min pace<br>- Cool Down / Stretch | - OFF | - OFF |
| **FRIDAY** | - OFF | **Complete 3 Rounds for Time**<br>- 10 Pull ups<br>- 25 Shoulder Circles (4 count)<br>- 30 Bicycles (4 count)<br>- 20 Swimmers<br>- 12 Dive Bombers<br>- 20 Rocky Sit ups<br>- 15 Bodyweight Rows<br>- 15 SHOULDER Pushups<br>- 15 Power Knees (each side)<br>- 15 Wide Pushups<br>- 8 Wide Pull ups<br>- 1 Minute Plank | **WARM UP:**<br>- 300m Freestyle<br>- 300m Lead arm- Trail arm, easy (fins)<br>**MAIN SET:**<br>- 3 x 100m Lead arm- Trail arm (fins), 95% effort, 2 min rest<br>- 3 x 200m Lead arm- Trail arm (fins), 85% effort, 2 min rest<br>- 2 x 500m Lead arm- Trail arm, 70% effort, 4 min rest<br>**COOL DOWN:** 100m Lead arm- Trail arm (fins), easy<br>**TOTAL: 2600m** |
| **SATURDAY** | - Dynamic Warm-up<br>- 5 1/2 Mile Run<br>  - Moderate Effort<br>- Cool Down / Stretch | OFF | OFF |
| **SUNDAY** | - OFF | OFF | OFF |

# PHASE 2 WORKOUT
## WEEK 6 OF 15

| | CARDIO | PHYSICAL TRAINING | SWIM |
|---|---|---|---|
| **MONDAY** | ○ OFF | **Complete 3 Rounds for Time**<br>7 PULL UPS<br>15 BODYWEIGHT TRICEPS EXTENSIONS<br>15 MODIFIED VSITS<br>15 BODYWEIGHT ROWS<br>20 DIPS<br>12 MOUNTAIN CLIMBERS (4 count)<br>5 WIDE PULL UPS<br>30 DIAMOND PUSHUPS<br>15 SIDE PLANK LEG LIFTS (each side)<br>10 FREEFALL ARCHES (5 SECONDS EACH)<br>12 SPHINX PUSHUPS<br>20 ROCKY SIT UPS | OFF |
| **TUESDAY** | ○ Dynamic Warm-up<br>○ 4 Mile Run<br>• Moderate Effort<br>○ Cool Down / Stretch | OFF | **WARM UP:**<br>○ 100m Freestyle<br>○ 100m Lead arm- Trail arm, easy (fins)<br>**MAIN SET:**<br>○ 3 x 100m Lead arm- Trail arm (fins), 95% effort, 3 min rest<br>○ 2 x 200m Lead arm- Trail arm (fins), 85% effort, 2 min rest<br>○ 1 x 500m Lead arm- Trail arm (fins), 70% effort, 1 min rest<br>**COOL DOWN:** 100m Lead arm- Trail arm (fins), easy<br>**TOTAL:** 1700m |
| **WEDNESDAY** | ○ OFF | **Complete 3 Rounds for Time**<br>○ 10 CHIN UPS<br>○ 15 SHOULDER PUSH UPS<br>○ 25 MODIFIED V-SITS<br>○ 15 UNDERHAND BODYWEIGHT ROWS<br>○ 8 WALL WALKS<br>○ 20 LEG RAISES<br>○ 12 BODYWEIGHT BICEP CURLS<br>○ 25 SHOULDER CIRCLES (4 count; EACH DIRECTION)<br>○ 15 LEG RAISES<br>○ 30 SECOND CHIN UP HOLD<br>○ 10 HANDSTAND PUSHUPS<br>○ 30 ARM FLUTTER KICKS (4 count) | **WARM UP:**<br>○ 300m Freestyle<br>○ 200m Lead arm- Trail arm, easy (fins)<br>**MAIN SET:**<br>○ 3 x 100m Lead arm- Trail arm , 95% effort, 3 min rest<br>○ 3 x 200m Lead arm- Trail arm (fins), 85% effort, 3 min rest<br>○ 2 x 500m Lead arm- Trail arm (fins), 70-80% effort, 2 min rest<br>**COOL DOWN:** 200m Lead arm- Trail arm , easy<br>**TOTAL:** 2600m |
| **THURSDAY** | ○ Dynamic Warm-up<br>○ Run 1 mile at 6:30 min pace, 4 min rest<br>○ Run 1 mile at 7:00 min pace, 4 min rest<br>○ Run 1 mile at 7:30 min pace<br>○ Cool Down / Stretch | ○ OFF | ○ OFF |
| **FRIDAY** | ○ OFF | **Complete 3 Rounds for Time**<br>○ 35 PUSHUPS<br>○ 25 AIR SQUATS<br>○ 15 V-UPS<br>○ 10 CORN COB PUSHUPS<br>○ 10 PLYO SPLIT SQUATS (4 count)<br>○ 30 FLUTTER KICKS (4 count)<br>○ 25 DECLINE PUSHUPS<br>○ 10 ONE LEG SQUATS<br>○ 20 POWER KNEES (each side)<br>○ 15 DIVE BOMBERS<br>○ 25 CALF RAISES<br>○ 40 BICYCLES (4 count) | **WARM UP:**<br>○ Freestyle<br>○ 200m Lead arm- Trail arm, easy (fins)<br>**MAIN SET:**<br>○ 3 x 100m Lead arm- Trail arm (fins), 95% effort, 3 min rest<br>○ 3 x 200m Lead arm- Trail arm (fins), 80% effort, 2 min rest<br>○ 1 x 500m Lead arm- Trail arm (fins), 70% effort, 30 sec rest<br>**COOL DOWN:** 200 m Lead arm- Trail arm , easy<br>**TOTAL:** 2000 m |
| **SATURDAY** | ○ Dynamic Warm-up<br>○ 3 Mile Run<br>• Low Effort<br>○ Cool Down / Stretch | ○ OFF | ○ OFF |
| **SUNDAY** | ○ OFF | ○ OFF | ○ OFF |

# PHASE 2 WORKOUT
## WEEK 7 OF 15

| | CARDIO | PHYSICAL TRAINING | SWIM |
|---|---|---|---|
| **MONDAY** | **PAST** <br> *Record 1.5 mi time for Interval Generator for re-calculation | **PAST** <br> * | **PAST** <br> * |
| **TUESDAY** | ○ OFF | **Complete 3 Rounds for Time** <br> ○ 15 DEEP SQUATS <br> ○ 15 SHOULDER PUSHUPS <br> ○ 40 FLUTTER KICKS (4 count) <br> ○ 10 ONE LEG SQUATS (each leg) <br> ○ 8 WALL WALKS <br> ○ 50 SIT UPS <br> ○ 10 SLIDING LEG CURLS (each leg) <br> ○ 10 HANDSTAND PUSHUPS <br> ○ 20 RUSSIAN TWISTS (4 count) <br> ○ 25 CALF RAISES (each leg) <br> ○ 25 SHOULDER CIRCLES (4 count) <br> ○ 20 POWER KNEES (each side) | **WARM UP:** <br> ○ 300m Freestyle <br> ○ 300m Lead arm- Trail arm, easy (fins) <br> **MAIN SET:** <br> ○ 3 x 100m Lead arm- Trail arm (fins), 95% effort, 1 min rest <br> ○ 3 x 200m Lead arm- Trail arm (fins), 85% effort, 3 min rest <br> ○ 1 x 500m Lead arm- Trail arm (fins), 70-80% effort, 2 min rest <br> **COOL DOWN:** 100 m Lead arm- Trail arm , easy <br> **TOTAL:** 2100 m |
| **WEDNESDAY** | ○ Dynamic Warm-up <br> ○ Interval Workout 1 <br>    • Reference Interval Generator for times <br> ○ Cool Down / Stretch | ○ OFF | **WARM UP:** <br> ○ 200m Freestyle <br> ○ 100m Lead arm- Trail arm, easy (fins) <br> **MAIN SET:** <br> ○ 2 x 100m Lead arm- Trail arm (fins), 95% effort, 1 min rest <br> ○ 2 x 200m Lead arm- Trail arm (fins), 85% effort, 1 min rest <br> ○ 1 x 500m Lead arm- Trail arm , 70-80% effort, 1 min rest <br> **COOL DOWN:** 100 m Lead arm- Trail arm (fins), easy <br> **TOTAL:** 1500 m |
| **THURSDAY** | ○ OFF | **AS MANY ROUNDS AS POSSIBLE (AMRAP) IN 20 MINUTES** <br> ○ 10 CHEST TO BAR PULL UPS <br> ○ 10 LEG RAISES <br> ○ 10 MOUNTAIN CLIMBERS (4 count) <br> ○ 10 CHIN UPS <br> ○ 10 RUSSIAN TWISTS (4 count) <br> ○ 10 PLYO SPLIT SQUAT | OFF |
| **FRIDAY** | ○ Dynamic Warm-up <br> ○ 6 Mile Run <br>    • Moderate Effort <br> ○ Cool Down / Stretch | **Complete 3 Rounds** <br> ○ 10 SQUAT JUMPS <br> ○ 20 PUSH UPS <br> ○ 15 PULL UPS <br> ○ WALKING LUNGE (5ea LEG) <br> ○ 10 DIPS <br> ○ 10 UNDERHAND BODYWEIGHT ROWS | **WARM UP:** <br> ○ 300m Freestyle <br> ○ 300m Lead arm- Trail arm, easy <br> **MAIN SET:** <br> ○ 3 x 100m Lead arm- Trail arm (fins), 95% effort, 2 min rest <br> ○ 3 x 200m Lead arm- Trail arm (fins), 85% effort, 2 min rest <br> ○ 2 x 500m Lead arm- Trail arm (fins), 70-80% effort, 3 min rest <br> **COOL DOWN:** 200 m Lead arm- Trail arm , easy <br> **TOTAL:** 2700 m |
| **SATURDAY** | ○ OFF | **Complete 3 Rounds for Time** <br> ○ 10 CHIN UPS <br> ○ 15 BODYWEIGHT TRICEPS EXTENSIONS <br> ○ 1 MINUTE PLANK <br> ○ 15 BODYWEIGHT BICEP CURLS <br> ○ 20 DIPS <br> ○ 10 MOUNTAIN CLIMBERS (4 count) <br> ○ 6 ONE ARM CHIN (EACH ARM) <br> ○ 15 SPHINX PUSHUPS <br> ○ 20 MODIFIED V-SITS <br> ○ 15 UNDERHAND BODYWEIGHT ROWS <br> ○ 25 DIAMOND PUSHUPS <br> ○ 30 SECOND SIDE PLANKS (each side) | OFF |
| **SUNDAY** | ○ OFF | OFF | OFF |

# PHASE 2 WORKOUT
## WEEK 8 OF 15

| | CARDIO | PHYSICAL TRAINING | SWIM |
|---|---|---|---|
| **MONDAY** | o Dynamic Warm-up<br><br>o Timed 3 ½ Mile<br>• Max Effort<br><br>o Cool Down / Stretch | Complete 3 Rounds for Time<br>o 40 PUSHUPS<br>o 35 AIR SQUATS<br>o 30 FLUTTER KICKS (4 count)<br>o 20 DECLINE PUSHUPS<br>o 10 PLYO SPLIT SQUATS (4 count)<br>o 20 MODIFIED V-SITS<br>o 15 DIVE BOMBERS<br>o 10 SLIDING LEG CURLS<br>o 15 MOUNTAIN CLIMBERS (4 count)<br>o 25 WIDE PUSHUPS<br>o 20 CALF RAISES (each leg)<br>o 1 MINUTE PLANK | o OFF |
| **TUESDAY** | o OFF | Complete 3 Rounds for Time<br>o 6 CHIN UPS<br>o 20 SHOULDER PUSHUPS<br>o 35 BICYCLES (4 count)<br>o 15 UNDERHAND BODYWEIGHT ROWS<br>o 10 CORN COB PUSHUPS<br>o 15 VUPS<br>o 7 NEGATIVE CHIN UPS<br>o 12 DIVE BOMBERS<br>o 15 HANGING LEG RAISES<br>o 15 BODYWEIGHT BICEP CURLS<br>o 5 WALL WALKS<br>o 15 POWER KNEES (each side) | **WARM UP:**<br>o 300m Freestyle<br>o 200m Lead arm- Trail arm, easy<br>**MAIN SET:**<br>o 1 x 200m Lead arm- Trail arm (fins), 85% effort, 1 min rest<br>o 2 x 600m Lead arm- Trail arm (fins), 70-80% effort, 4 min rest<br>**COOL DOWN:** 100m Lead arm- Trail arm, easy<br>**TOTAL:** 2000m |
| **WEDNESDAY** | o Dynamic Warm-up<br><br>o Interval Workout 2<br>• Reference Interval Generator for times<br><br>o Cool Down / Stretch | o OFF | **WARM UP:**<br>o 300m Freestyle<br>o 300m Lead arm- Trail arm, easy<br>**MAIN SET:**<br>o 2 x 200m Lead arm- Trail arm (fins), 85% effort, 2 min rest<br>o 3 x 600m Lead arm- Trail arm (fins), 70% effort, 2 min rest<br>**COOL DOWN:** 200m Lead arm- Trail arm, easy<br>**TOTAL:** 3000m |
| **THURSDAY** | o OFF | Complete 3 Rounds for Time<br>o 30 DIAMOND PUSHUPS<br>o 12 PULL UPS<br>o 40 BICYCLES (4 count)<br>o 20 DIPS<br>o 15 BODYWEIGHT ROWS<br>o 20 LEG RAISES<br>o 15 SPHINX PUSHUPS<br>o 10 5 SECOND FREEFALL ARCHES<br>o 30 SECOND LSITS<br>o 15 BODYWEIGHT TRICEPS EXTENSIONS<br>o 6 WIDE PULL UPS<br>o 45 SIT UPS | o OFF |
| **FRIDAY** | o Dynamic Warm-up<br>o 6 Mile Run<br>• Moderate Effort<br>o Cool Down / Stretch | **Complete 3 Rounds**<br>o 15 AIR SQUATS<br>o 30 SECOND FOREARM PLANK<br>o 10 BURPEES<br>o SIDE LUNGES (5ea LEG)<br>o 30 SECOND SIDE PLANK (each side)<br>o 10 SQUAT JUMPS<br>o 5 TOES TO BAR | o OFF |
| **SATURDAY** | o OFF | **AS MANY ROUNDS AS POSSIBLE (AMRAP) IN 20 MINUTES**<br>o 10 CHEST TO BAR PULL UPS<br>o 10 LEG RAISES<br>o 10 MOUNTAIN CLIMBERS (4 count)<br>o 10 CHIN UPS<br>o 10 RUSSIAN TWISTS (4 count)<br>o 10 PLYO SPLIT SQUAT | **WARM UP:**<br>o 200m Freestyle<br>o 100m Lead arm- Trail arm, easy<br>**MAIN SET:**<br>o 2 x 200m Lead arm- Trail arm (fins), 85% effort, 2 min rest<br>o 2 x 600m Lead arm- Trail arm (fins), 75% effort, 3 min rest<br>**COOL DOWN:** 100m Lead arm- Trail arm (fins), easy<br>**TOTAL:** 2000m |
| **SUNDAY** | o OFF | o OFF | o OFF |

# PHASE 2 WORKOUT
## WEEK 9 OF 15

| | CARDIO | PHYSICAL TRAINING | SWIM |
|---|---|---|---|
| **MONDAY** | ○ Dynamic Warm-up<br>○ Timed 3 ¾ Mile<br>• Max Effort<br>○ Cool Down / Stretch | **Complete 3 Rounds for Time**<br>15 PULL UPS<br>15 BODYWEIGHT TRICEPS EXTENSIONS<br>20 MODIFIED VSITS<br>6 EXPLOSIVE PULL UPS WITH GRIP SWITCH<br>15 SPHINX PUSHUPS<br>25 POWER KNEES (each side)<br>20 BODYWEIGHT ROWS<br>20 DIAMOND PUSHUPS<br>45 SECOND SIDE PLANKS (each side)<br>20 SWIMMERS<br>25 DIPS<br>30 FLUTTER KICKS (4 count) | ○ OFF |
| **TUESDAY** | ○ OFF | **Complete 3 Rounds for Time**<br>40 PUSHUPS<br>15 CHIN UPS<br>15 CAN CAN ABS<br>15 DIVE BOMBERS<br>15 BODYWEIGHT BICEP CURLS<br>30 FLUTTER KICKS (4 count)<br>35 DECLINE PUSHUPS<br>15 UNDERHAND BODYWEIGHT ROWS<br>20 POWER KNEES (each side)<br>15 DIVE BOMBERS<br>5 ONE ARM CHIN UPS (EACH ARM)<br>1 MINUTE PLANK | **WARM UP:**<br>○ 200m Freestyle<br>○ 100m Lead arm- Trail arm, easy<br>**MAIN SET:**<br>○ 2 x 200m Lead arm- Trail arm (fins), 85% effort, 2 min rest<br>○ 3 x 600m Lead arm- Trail arm (fins), 75% effort, 3 min rest<br>**COOL DOWN:** 100m Lead arm- Trail arm, easy<br>**TOTAL:** 2600m |
| **WEDNESDAY** | ○ Dynamic Warm-up<br>○ Interval Workout 3<br>• Reference Interval Generator for times<br>○ Cool Down / Stretch | ○ OFF | ○ OFF |
| **THURSDAY** | ○ OFF | **3 Rounds for Time**<br>○ 20 METER BEAR CRAWL<br>○ 25 SQUAT<br>○ 20 METER CRAB CRAWL<br>○ 10 REVERSE LUNGE (each side)<br>○ 10 METER INCHWORM<br>○ 15 DIAMOND PUSH UP | **WARM UP:**<br>○ 300m Freestyle<br>○ 300m Lead arm- Trail arm, easy<br>**MAIN SET:**<br>○ 2 x 200m Lead arm- Trail arm (fins), 85% effort, 2 min rest<br>○ 3 x 600m Lead arm- Trail arm (fins), 70-80% effort, 3 min rest<br>**COOL DOWN:** 100m Lead arm- Trail arm, easy<br>**TOTAL:** 2900m |
| **FRIDAY** | ○ Dynamic Warm-up<br>○ 6 Mile Run<br>• Moderate Effort<br>○ Cool Down / Stretch | **Complete 3 Rounds for Time**<br>○ 15 SHOULDER PUSHUPS<br>○ 10 PLYO SPLIT SQUATS (4 count)<br>○ 20 V-UPS<br>○ 20 SHOULDER CIRCLES (4 count; EACH DIRECTION)<br>○ 25 BODY SQUATS<br>○ 12 MOUNTAIN CLIMBERS (4 count)<br>○ 8 WALL WALKS<br>○ 12 SLIDING LEG CURLS (each leg)<br>○ 35 BICYCLES (4 count)<br>○ 10 HANDSTAND PUSHUPS<br>○ 25 CALF RAISES (each leg)<br>○ 30 FLUTTER KICKS (4 count) | ○ OFF |
| **SATURDAY** | ○ OFF | **5 Rounds for Time**<br>○ 20 AIR SQUATS<br>○ 20 PUSH UPS<br>○ ALTERNATING LUNGES (10ea LEG)<br>○ 10 SUPERMANS<br>○ 10 V-UPS | **WARM UP:**<br>○ 100m Freestyle<br>○ 100m Lead arm- Trail arm, easy (fins)<br>**MAIN SET:**<br>○ 2 x 200m Lead arm- Trail arm (fins), 85% effort, 1 min rest<br>○ 1 x 600m Lead arm- Trail arm (fins), 70-80% effort, 1 min rest<br>**COOL DOWN:** 200m Lead arm- Trail arm (fins), easy<br>**TOTAL:** 1400 m |
| **SUNDAY** | ○ OFF | ○ OFF | ○ OFF |

# PHASE 2 WORKOUT
## WEEK 10 OF 15

|   | CARDIO | PHYSICAL TRAINING | SWIM |
|---|---|---|---|
| **MONDAY** | - Dynamic Warm-up<br>- Timed 4 Mile<br>  - Max Effort<br>- Cool Down / Stretch | Complete 3 Rounds for Time<br>- 12 PULL UPS<br>- 40 PUSHUPS<br>- 15 RUSSIAN TWISTS (4 count)<br>- 8 WIDE PULL UPS<br>- 25 WIDE PUSHUPS<br>- 35 BICYCLES (4 count)<br>- 20 BODYWEIGHT ROWS<br>- 10 DIVE BOMBERS<br>- 35 FLUTTER KICKS (4 count)<br>- 10 SUPERMANS<br>- 30 DECLINE PUSHUPS<br>- 20 LEG LIFTS | - OFF |
| **TUESDAY** | - OFF | - OFF | **WARM UP:**<br>- Freestyle<br>- 100m Lead arm- Trail arm, easy<br>**MAIN SET:**<br>- 2 x 200m Lead arm- Trail arm (fins), 85% effort, 1 min rest<br>- 3 x 600m Lead arm- Trail arm , 70-80% effort, 2 min rest<br>**COOL DOWN:** 200m Lead arm- Trail arm (fins), easy<br>**TOTAL:** 2700m |
| **WEDNESDAY** | - Dynamic Warm-up<br>- Interval Workout 4<br>  - Reference Interval Generator for times<br>- Cool Down / Stretch | Complete 3 Rounds for Time<br>- 15 SHOULDER PUSHUPS<br>- 15 CHIN UPS<br>- 10 JUMPING JACKS (4 count)<br>- 25 ARM FLUTTER KICKS (4 count)<br>- 15 UNDERHAND BODYWEIGHT ROWS<br>- 15 MOUNTAIN CLIMBERS (4 count)<br>- 10 HANDSTAND PUSHUPS<br>- 15 UNDERHAND BODYWEIGHT ROWS<br>- 15 RUSSIAN TWISTS (4 count)<br>- 20 SHOULDER CIRCLES (4 count; each direction)<br>- 4 ONE ARM CHIN UPS (Each arm)<br>- 20 POWER KNEES (each side) | - OFF |
| **THURSDAY** | - OFF | - OFF | **WARM UP:**<br>- 300m Freestyle<br>- 300m Lead arm- Trail arm, easy<br>**MAIN SET:**<br>- 2 x 200m Lead arm- Trail arm (fins), 85% effort, 1 min rest<br>- 3 x 600m Lead arm- Trail arm (fins), 70% effort, 3 min rest<br>**COOL DOWN:** 200m Lead arm- Trail arm (fins), easy<br>**TOTAL:** 3000m |
| **FRIDAY** | - Dynamic Warm-up<br>- 6 Mile Run<br>  - Moderate Effort<br>- Cool Down / Stretch | **COMPLETE 3 ROUNDS FOR TIME**<br>- 12 PLYO SPLIT SQUATS (4 count)<br>- 30 DIAMOND PUSHUPS<br>- 20 CAN CAN ABS<br>- 25 CALF RAISES (each leg)<br>- 20 DIPS<br>- 30 BICYCLES (4 count)<br>- 10 ONE LEG SQUATS (each leg)<br>- 12 SPHINX PUSHUPS<br>- 10 MOUNTAIN CLIMBERS (4 count)<br>- 12 SWISS BALL LEG CURLS (each leg)<br>- 15 BODYWEIGHT TRICEPS EXTENSIONS<br>- 20 MODIFIED VSITS | - OFF |
| **SATURDAY** | - OFF | - OFF | **WARM UP:**<br>- 100m Freestyle<br>- 100m Lead arm- Trail arm, easy<br>**MAIN SET:**<br>- 2 x 600m Lead arm- Trail arm (fins), 70-80% effort, 30 sec rest<br>**COOL DOWN:** 200m Lead arm- Trail arm (fins), easy<br>**TOTAL:** 1600m |
| **SUNDAY** | - OFF | - OFF | - OFF |

# PHASE 2 WORKOUT
## WEEK 11 OF 15

| | CARDIO | PHYSICAL TRAINING | SWIM |
|---|---|---|---|
| **MONDAY** | ○ Dynamic Warm-up<br>○ Timed 3 ½ Mile<br>• Max Effort<br>○ Cool Down / Stretch | **COMPLETE 3 ROUNDS FOR TIME**<br>○ 40 DECLINE PUSHUPS<br>○ 5 ONE ARM CHIN UPS (EACH ARM)<br>○ 30 UNSUPPORTED SIT UPS<br>○ 45 PUSHUPS<br>○ 10 BODYWEIGHT BICEP CURLS<br>○ 20 SIDE PLANK LEG LIFTS<br>○ 10 CORN COB PUSHUPS<br>○ 15 CHIN UPS<br>○ 40 FLUTTER KICKS (4 count)<br>○ 25 WIDE PUSHUPS<br>○ 20 UNDERHAND BODYWEIGHT ROWS<br>○ 25 MODIFIED V-SITS | ○ OFF |
| **TUESDAY** | ○ OFF | ○ OFF | ○ OFF |
| **WEDNESDAY** | ○ Dynamic Warm-up<br>○ Interval Workout 5<br>• Reference Interval Generator for times<br>○ Cool Down / Stretch | **Complete 3 Rounds for Time**<br>○ 15 DIVE BOMBERS<br>○ 25 AIR SQUATS<br>○ 40 BICYCLES (4 count)<br>○ 10 CORN COB PUSHUPS<br>○ 15 PLYO SPLIT SQUATS (4 count)<br>○ 1 MINUTE 30 SECOND PLANK<br>○ 8 WALL WALKS<br>○ 15 DONKEY KICKS (each leg)<br>○ 15 RUSSIAN TWISTS (4 count)<br>○ 25 SHOULDER CIRCLES (each direction)<br>○ 25 CALF RAISES (each leg)<br>○ 30 SECOND L-SIT | **WARM UP:**<br>○ 400m Freestyle<br>○ 400m Lead arm- Trail arm, easy<br>**MAIN SET:**<br>○ 3 x 200m Lead arm- Trail arm (fins), 85% effort, 2 min rest<br>○ 2 x 700m Lead arm- Trail arm (fins), 70% effort, 3 min rest<br>**COOL DOWN:** 200m Lead arm- Trail arm, easy<br>**TOTAL:** 3000m |
| **THURSDAY** | ○ OFF | ○ OFF | ○ OFF |
| **FRIDAY** | ○ Dynamic Warm-up<br>○ 6 Mile Run<br>• Moderate Effort<br>○ Cool Down / Stretch | **Complete 3 Rounds for Time**<br>○ 15 PULL UPS<br>○ 15 BODYWEIGHT TRICEPS EXTENSIONS<br>○ 20 MODIFIED V-SITS<br>○ 20 BODYWEIGHT ROWS<br>○ 20 DIPS<br>○ 50 FLUTTER KICKS (4 count)<br>○ 6 ONE ARM PULL UPS<br>○ 35 DIAMOND PUSHUPS<br>○ 35 BICYCLES (4 count)<br>○ 12 SUPERMANS<br>○ 15 SPHINX PUSHUPS<br>○ 20 POWER KNEES (each side) | ○ OFF |
| **SATURDAY** | ○ OFF | ○ OFF | **WARM UP:**<br>○ 300m Freestyle<br>○ 200m Lead arm- Trail arm, easy (fins)<br>**MAIN SET:**<br>○ 2 x 700m Lead arm- Trail arm (fins), 70% effort, 2 min rest<br>○ 3 x 200m Lead arm- Trail arm (fins), 85% effort, 1 min rest<br>**COOL DOWN:** 200m Lead arm- Trail arm, easy<br>**TOTAL:** 2700m |
| **SUNDAY** | ○ OFF | ○ OFF | ○ OFF |

# PHASE 2 WORKOUT
## WEEK 12 OF 15

| | CARDIO | PHYSICAL TRAINING | SWIM |
|---|---|---|---|
| **MONDAY** | - Dynamic Warm-up<br>- Timed 3 ½ Mile<br>  - Max Effort<br>- Cool Down / Stretch | **Complete 3 Rounds for Time**<br>- 15 DIPS<br>- 30 SECOND CHIN UP HOLDS<br>- 20 MODIFIED V-SITS<br>- 30 DIAMOND PUSHUPS<br>- 15 CHIN UPS<br>- 30 BICYCLES (4 count)<br>- 10 SPHINX PUSHUPS<br>- 15 UNDERHAND BODYWEIGHT ROWS<br>- 15 RUSSIAN TWISTS (4 count)<br>- 15 BODYWEIGHT TRICEPS EXTENSIONS<br>- 4 ONE ARM CHIN UPS (EACH ARM)<br>- 20 POWER KNEES (each side) | - OFF |
| **TUESDAY** | - OFF | **Complete 3 Rounds**<br>- 15 AIR SQUATS<br>- 30 SECOND FOREARM PLANK<br>- 10 BURPEES<br>- SIDE LUNGES (5ea LEG)<br>- 30 SECOND SIDE PLANK (each side)<br>- 10 SQUAT JUMPS<br>- 5 TOES TO BAR | **WARM UP:**<br>- 200m Freestyle<br>- 200m Lead arm- Trail arm, easy<br>**MAIN SET:**<br>- 3 x 200m Lead arm- Trail arm (fins), 85% effort, 2 min rest<br>- 2 x 700m Lead arm- Trail arm (fins), 70-80% effort, 2 min rest<br>**COOL DOWN:** 200m Lead arm- Trail arm, easy<br>**TOTAL: 2600m** |
| **WEDNESDAY** | **AM**<br>- Dynamic Warm-up<br>- Interval Workout 6<br>  - Reference Interval Generator for times<br>- Cool Down / Stretch | **Complete 3 Rounds for Time**<br>- 15 SHOULDER PUSHUPS<br>- 12 PULL UPS<br>- 20 RUSSIAN TWISTS (4 count)<br>- 25 SHOULDER CIRCLES (4 count; EACH DIRECTION)<br>- 8 WIDE PULL UPS<br>- 20 POWER KNEES (each side)<br>- 30 ARM FLUTTER KICKS (4 count)<br>- 20 SWIMMERS<br>- 10 MOUNTAIN CLIMBERS (4 count)<br>- 12 DIVE BOMBERS<br>- 15 BODYWEIGHT ROWS<br>- 20 MODIFIED VSITS | - OFF |
| **THURSDAY** | - OFF | - OFF | **WARM UP:**<br>- 400m Freestyle<br>- 400m Lead arm- Trail arm, easy<br>**MAIN SET:**<br>- 3 x 200m Lead arm- Trail arm, 85% effort, 20 sec rest<br>- 2 x 700m Lead arm- Trail arm, 70% effort, 30 sec rest<br>**COOL DOWN:** 200m Lead arm- Trail arm, easy<br>**TOTAL: 3000m** |
| **FRIDAY** | - Dynamic Warm-up<br>- 6 Mile Run<br>  - Moderate Effort<br>- Cool Down / Stretch | **AS MANY ROUNDS AS POSSIBLE (AMRAP) IN 20 MINUTES**<br>- 5 PULL UPS<br>- 10 PUSH UPS<br>- 15 AIR SQUATS | - OFF |
| **SATURDAY** | - OFF | **Complete 3 Rounds for Time**<br>- 35 DECLINE PUSHUPS<br>- 20 DEEP SQUATS<br>- 30 UNSUPPORTED SIT UPS<br>- 40 PUSHUPS<br>- 10 PLYO SPLIT SQUATS (4 count)<br>- 1 MINUTE 30 SECOND PLANK<br>- 10 CORN COB PUSHUPS<br>- 25 METER CRABWALK<br>- 40 FLUTTER KICKS (4 count)<br>- 15 CLAPPING PUSHUPS<br>- 25 CALF RAISES (each leg)<br>- 15 V-UPS | **WARM UP:**<br>- 100m Freestyle<br>- 100m Lead arm- Trail arm, easy<br>**MAIN SET:**<br>- 2 x 700m Lead arm- Trail arm (fins), 70-80% effort, 30 sec rest<br>**COOL DOWN:** 200m Lead arm- Trail arm (fins), easy<br>**TOTAL: 1000m** |
| **SUNDAY** | - OFF | - OFF | - OFF |

# PHASE 2 WORKOUT
## WEEK 13 OF 15

| | CARDIO | PHYSICAL TRAINING | SWIM |
|---|---|---|---|
| **MONDAY** | - Dynamic Warm-up<br>- Timed 3 Mile<br>  - Max Effort<br>- Cool Down / Stretch | **Complete 3 Rounds**<br>- 10 SQUAT JUMPS<br>- 20 PUSH UPS<br>- 15 PULL UPS<br>- WALKING LUNGE (5ea LEG)<br>- 10 DIPS<br>- 10 UNDERHAND BODYWEIGHT ROWS | - OFF |
| **TUESDAY** | - OFF | **Complete 3 Rounds for Time**<br>- 15 PLYO PUSH UP<br>- 15 PLYO SPLIT SQUAT (each leg)<br>- 15 L-SIT PULL UP<br>- 30 SECOND PLANK<br>- 10 JUMP SQUATS | **WARM UP:**<br>- 200m Freestyle<br>- 100m Lead arm- Trail arm, easy<br>**MAIN SET:**<br>- 2 x 200m Lead arm- Trail arm, 85% effort, 1 min rest<br>- 2 x 700m Lead arm- Trail arm (fins), 70-80% effort, 2 min rest<br>**COOL DOWN:** 100 m Lead arm- Trail arm (fins), easy<br>**TOTAL:** 2200 m |
| **WEDNESDAY** | - Dynamic Warm-up<br>- Interval Workout 7<br>  - Reference Interval Generator for times<br>- Cool Down / Stretch | - OFF | **WARM UP:**<br>- 400m Freestyle<br>- 400m Lead arm- Trail arm, easy (fins)<br>**MAIN SET:**<br>- 3 x 200m Lead arm- Trail arm (fins), 85% effort, 20 sec rest<br>- 1 x 700m Lead arm- Trail arm , 70-80% effort, 30 sec rest<br>**COOL DOWN:** 200m Lead arm- Trail arm , easy<br>**TOTAL:** 2300m |
| **THURSDAY** | - OFF | - OFF | - OFF |
| **FRIDAY** | - Dynamic Warm-up<br>- 6 Mile Run<br>  - Moderate Effort<br>- Cool Down / Stretch | **AMRAP 20 minutes**<br>- 10 JUMP SQUAT<br>- 10 PLYO PUSH<br>- 10 PLYO SPLIT SQUAT<br>- 10 SINGLE LEG GLUTE BRIDGE (each leg)<br>- 10 WIDE PUSH UPS | **WARM UP:**<br>- 400m Freestyle<br>- 400m Lead arm- Trail arm, easy (fins)<br>**MAIN SET:**<br>- 3 x 200m Lead arm- Trail arm (fins), 85% effort, 1 min rest<br>- 2 x 700m Lead arm- Trail arm (fins), 70% effort, 2 min rest<br>**COOL DOWN:** 200 m Lead arm- Trail arm , easy<br>**TOTAL:** 3000 m |
| **SATURDAY** | - OFF | **Complete 1 Round**<br>- ½ MILE JOG WARMUP<br>- ALTERNATE NEXT TWO EXERCISES UNTIL A TOTAL OF 800 METERS IS REACHED<br>- 100 METER SPRINT<br>- 100 METER LUNGE WALK<br><br>- 100 PULLUPS AS MANY SETS AS NECESSARY<br>- 800 METER RUN<br>- 75 VUPS<br>- 75 HANGING KNEES TO ELBOWS<br>- 800 METER COOL DOWN | - OFF |
| **SUNDAY** | - OFF | - OFF | - OFF |

# PHASE 2 WORKOUT
## WEEK 14 OF 15

|  | CARDO | PHYSICAL TRAINING | SWIM |
|---|---|---|---|
| **MONDAY** | - Dynamic Warm-up<br>- Timed 3 Mile<br>  - Max Effort<br>- Cool Down / Stretch | - OFF | - OFF |
| **TUESDAY** | - OFF | **Complete 3 Rounds for Time**<br>- 15 CHIN UPS<br>- 20 BODYWEIGHT TRICEPS EXTENSIONS<br>- 20 MODIFIED V-SITS<br>- 15 UNDERHAND BODYWEIGHT ROWS<br>- 20 DIPS<br>- 50 FLUTTER KICKS (4 count)<br>- 15 BODYWEIGHT BICEP CURLS<br>- 35 DIAMOND PUSHUPS<br>- 35 BICYCLES (4 count)<br>- 45 SECOND CHIN UP HOLD<br>- 10 SPHINX PUSHUPS<br>- 20 POWER KNEES (each side) | **WARM UP:**<br>- 200m Freestyle<br>- 200m Lead arm- Trail arm, easy<br>**MAIN SET:**<br>- 1 x 1500m Lead arm- Trail arm (fins), 70-80% effort<br>**COOL DOWN:** 100m Lead arm- Trail arm, easy<br>**TOTAL:** 2000m |
| **WEDNESDAY** | - Dynamic Warm-up<br>- Interval Workout 8<br>  - Reference Interval Generator for times<br>- Cool Down / Stretch | - OFF | - OFF |
| **THURSDAY** | - OFF | **Complete 3 Rounds for Time**<br>- 45 PUSHUPS<br>- 15 PULL UPS<br>- 40 BICYCLES (4 count)<br>- 35 DECLINE PUSHUPS<br>- 15 BODYWEIGHT ROWS<br>- 1 MINUTE 30 SECOND PLANK<br>- 20 CLAPPING PUSHUPS<br>- 8 WIDE PULL UPS<br>- 40 FLUTTER KICKS (4 count)<br>- 20 JUMPING JACKS (4 count)<br>- 10 SUPERMANS<br>- 25 MODIFIED V-SITS | - OFF |
| **FRIDAY** | - Dynamic Warm-up<br>- 6 Mile Run<br>  - Moderate Effort<br>- Cool Down / Stretch | - OFF | **WARM UP:**<br>- 300m Freestyle<br>- 300m Lead arm- Trail arm, easy<br>**MAIN SET:**<br>- 1 x 2000m Lead arm- Trail arm (fins), 70-80% effort<br>**COOL DOWN:** 200m Lead arm- Trail arm, easy<br>**TOTAL:** 2800m |
| **SATURDAY** | - OFF | **Complete 3 Rounds for Time**<br>- 30 AIR SQUATS<br>- 15 SHOULDER PUSHUPS<br>- 30 UNSUPPORTED SIT UPS<br>- 10 TWISTING LUNGES (each leg)<br>- 6 WALL WALKS<br>- 1 MINUTE 45 SECOND PLANK<br>- 12 GLUTE HAM RAISE<br>- 12 HANDSTAND PUSHUPS<br>- 20 RUSSIAN TWISTS (4 count)<br>- 25 CALF RAISES (each leg)<br>- 25 SHOULDER CIRCLES (4 count; each direction)<br>- 20 POWER KNEES (each side) | - OFF |
| **SUNDAY** | - OFF | - OFF | - OFF |

# PHASE 2 WORKOUT
## WEEK 15 OF 15

| | CARDIO | PHYSICAL TRAINING | SWIM |
|---|---|---|---|
| **MONDAY** | *Start at Physical Training, then run, then Swim<br>o Dynamic Warm-up<br><br>o Timed 3 Mile for time<br>• Max Effort<br><br>o Cool Down – 30 Minute rest before swim | o Dynamic warm-up<br>o Max effort pull ups in 1minute<br>o Max effort sit ups in 2 minutes<br>o Max effort pushups in 2 minutes<br>o Cool down – 10 minute rest before run | o Dynamic Warm-up<br><br>o Timed 1500 meter<br>• Max Effort<br><br>o Cool Down / Stretch |
| **TUESDAY** | o OFF | **5 Rounds for Time**<br>o 20 PULL UPS<br>o 30 PUSH UPS<br>o 40 SIT UPS<br>o 50 AIR SQUATS<br><br>REST 3 MINUTES BETWEEN ROUNDS ADD TIMES FROM EACH ROUND TO GET TOTAL TIME | **WARM UP:**<br>o 300m Freestyle<br>o 300m Lead arm- Trail arm, easy<br>**MAIN SET:**<br>o 1 x 1800m Lead arm- Trail arm (fins), 70% effort<br>**COOL DOWN:** 100m Lead arm- Trail arm, easy<br>**TOTAL:** 2500m |
| **WEDNESDAY** | o Dynamic Warm-up<br>o Run 1 mile at 6:45 min pace<br>o Rest for 4 min<br>o Run 2 miles at 7:30 min pace, rest 5 min<br>o Run 1 mile at 7:00 min pace<br>o Cool Down / Stretch | o OFF | o OFF |
| **THURSDAY** | o OFF | **AS MANY ROUNDS AS POSSIBLE (AMRAP) IN 20 MINUTES**<br>o 10 CHEST TO BAR PULL UPS<br>o 10 LEG RAISES<br>o 10 MOUNTAIN CLIMBERS (4 count)<br>o 10 CHIN UPS<br>o 10 RUSSIAN TWISTS (4 count)<br>o 10 PLYO SPLIT SQUAT | **PM**<br>**WARM UP:**<br>o 200m Freestyle<br>o 200m Lead arm- Trail arm, easy<br>**MAIN SET:**<br>o 1 x 2200m Lead arm- Trail arm (fins), 70-80% effort<br>**COOL DOWN:** 200m Lead arm- Trail arm, easy<br>**TOTAL:** 2800m |
| **FRIDAY** | o Dynamic Warm-up<br>o 6 Mile Run<br>• Moderate Effort<br>o Cool Down / Stretch | o OFF | o OFF |
| **SATURDAY** | o OFF | **Complete 3 Rounds for Time**<br>o 20 PULL UPS<br>o 20 BODYWEIGHT TRICEPS EXTENSIONS<br>o 10 SCORPIONS (each side)<br>o 20 BODYWEIGHT ROWS<br>o 40 DIPS<br>o 50 BICYCLES (4 count)<br>o 15 EXPLOSIVE PULL UPS WITH GRIP SWITCH<br>o 50 FLUTTER KICKS (4 count)<br>o 15 FRONT LEVERS<br>o 40 DIAMOND PUSHUPS<br>o 25 LEG RAISES | **WARM UP:**<br>o 100m Freestyle<br>o 100m Lead arm- Trail arm, easy<br>**MAIN SET:**<br>o 1 x 1600m Lead arm- Trail arm (fins), 70-80% effort<br>**COOL DOWN:** 200m Lead arm- Trail arm, easy<br>**TOTAL:** 2000m |
| **SUNDAY** | o OFF | o OFF | o OFF |

Made in the USA
Las Vegas, NV
13 May 2025